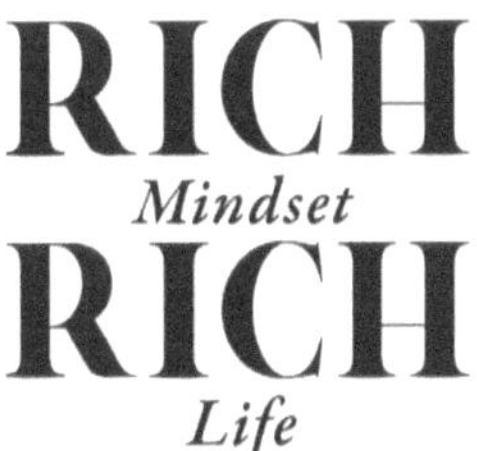

Napoleon Hill (1883–1970), best known for his global bestseller *Think and Grow Rich*, was a self-help author and businessman whose work has influenced millions across the world.

James Allen (1864–1912) retired from the business world to pursue a lifestyle of contemplation and wrote many books, including *As a Man Thinketh* and *The Path of Prosperity*.

Dale Harbison Carnegie (1888–1955), the bestselling author of *How to Win Friends and Influence People*, was an American writer and creator of famous courses in self-development, public speaking and interpersonal skills.

Roger Fritz (1928–2011) was an American management consultant and the author of over 63 self-help and management development books, including *The Power of a Positive Attitude* and *What Managers Need to Know*.

RICH *Mindset*
RICH *Life*

Transforming Your Finances and Future

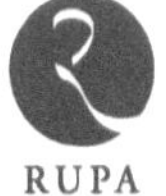

RUPA

Published by
Rupa Publications India Pvt. Ltd 2024
7/16, Ansari Road, Daryaganj
New Delhi 110002

Sales centres:
Bengaluru Chennai
Hyderabad Jaipur Kathmandu
Kolkata Mumbai Prayagraj

Edition copyright © Rupa Publications India Pvt. Ltd 2024

P-ISBN: 978-93-5702-798-4
E-ISBN: 978-93-5702-996-4

First impression 2024

10 9 8 7 6 5 4 3 2 1

Printed in India

CONTENTS

1

THE BEGINNING OF ALL RICHES

Napoleon Hill

The Largest Audience ever assembled in the history of mankind sat breathlessly awaiting the message of a mysterious man who was about to reveal to the world the secret of his riches.

In that audience were men who had tried and failed so often that they had all but lost hope!

And there were young men and young women—mere boys and girls—who were filled with hope and courage and eagerness to learn the way to riches.

There were doctors, lawyers, dentists, engineers and school teachers, waiting to hear what the speaker might have to say which would put them on the road to riches.

Clergymen of every religion on earth were there, with the hope that they might gather from the message of the speaker some inspirational ideas they could pass on to the members of their congregations.

Newspaper reporters were more numerous than bees; a great battery of cameras trained upon the speaker's platform, and the newsreel men were present with their moving picture cameras and sound equipment.

There were taxicab drivers, mechanics, bricklayers, merchants, barbers, and newsboys, representing every trade and every calling on earth, and many of them had come from distant places.

Slowly the curtain began to rise, the Chairman walking to the speaker's dais raised his hand for silence! The noise died down and a silent hush spread over the great audience.

The introduction of the speaker was brief. The Chairman simply said, "Ladies and Gentlemen, I have the honor to introduce to you the richest man in all the world. He has come to tell you about the MASTER-KEY TO RICHES."

The speaker walked briskly to the speaker's dais.

He was dressed in a long black robe and wore a mask over his eyes.

His hair was of a grayish tint, and he appeared to be about sixty years of age.

He stood silently for a few moments, while the cameras flashed. Then, speaking slowly, in a voice soft and pleasing, like music, he began his message:

You have come here to seek the MASTER-KEY TO RICHES!

You have come because of that human urge for the better things in life, which is the common desire of all people.

You desire economic security which money alone can provide.

Some of you desire an outlet for your talents in order that you may have the joy of creating your own riches.

Some of you are seeking the easy way to riches, with the hope that you will find it without giving anything in return; that too is a common desire. But it is a desire I shall hope to modify for your benefit, as from experience I have learned that there is no such thing as something for nothing.

THE MAGIC POTION THAT LEADS TO RICHES

This MASTER-KEY is an ingenious device with which those who possess it may unlock the door to the solution of all of their problems. Its powers of magic transcend those of the famous Aladdin's Lamp.

It opens the door to sound health.

It opens the door to love and romance.

It opens the door to friendship, by revealing the traits of personality and character which make enduring friends.

It reveals the method by which every adversity, every failure, every disappointment, every mistaken error of judgment, and every past defeat may be transmuted into riches of a priceless value.

It kindles anew the dead hopes of all who possess it, and it reveals the formula by which one may "tune in" and draw upon the great reservoir of Infinite Intelligence, through that state of mind known as Faith.

It lifts humble men to positions of power, fame and fortune.

It turns back the hands of the clock of Time and renews the spirit of youth for those who have grown old too soon.

It provides the method by which one may take full and complete possession of one's own mind, thus giving one unchallengeable control over the emotions of the heart and the power of thinking.

It bridges the deficiencies of those who have inadequate education through formal schooling, and puts them substantially on the same plane of opportunity that is enjoyed by those who have a better education.

And lastly, it opens the doors, one by one, to the Twelve Great Riches of Life, which I shall presently describe for you in detail.

Listen carefully to what I have to say, for I shall not pass this way again. Listen not only with open ears, but with open minds and eager hearts, remembering that no man may hear that for which he has not the preparation for hearing.

The preparation consists of many things, among them sincerity of purpose, humility of heart, a full recognition of the truth that no man knows everything; that the combined knowledge of mankind has not been enough to save men from cutting one another to pieces through warfare, nor to restrain them from cheating and stealing the fruits of labor from their fellowmen.

I shall speak to you of facts and describe to you many principles of which many of you may never have heard, for they are known only to those who have prepared themselves to accept the MASTER-KEY—a small but ever-increasing number of people who have attained the Degree of Fellowship.

The Fellowship is made up of men and women from many walks of life, of all nationalities and creeds. Its purpose is to reveal to mankind the benefits which are available through the spirit of the Brotherhood of man.

The Fellowship was born of the necessity of rehabilitating a war-worn world into which civilization was brought to the very brink of destruction through World War II. The Fellowship is non-sectarian and noncommercial.

Its members work individually. It has no authorized leaders, but every one who qualifies for the Degree of Fellowship becomes a leader unto himself.

The only condition that is required for membership is that all who qualify for the degree shall share with others the benefits they receive through the MASTER-KEY TO RICHES—as many others as they may find who are willing to prepare themselves to receive the benefits.

The Fellowship prepares men and women to relate themselves to one another as brothers and sisters.

It recognizes the great abundance of material riches available for mankind and provides a rational plan by which every person may share in these riches in proportion to his talents, as they are expressed through useful service.

It frowns upon the idea of too much for the few and too little for the many, but it also discourages all who endeavor to get something for nothing. And it discourages the accumulation of riches by individuals whose greed inspires them to seek more than they can use for their own economic security and to provide opportunities through which others may attain such security.

The Fellowship has a stupendous task ahead of it.

Civilization must live and go forward, not backward, for that is the plan of the Creator of all things.

Men must learn to live together as brothers, so that they may walk arm in arm, do the world's work and reap their just reward without poverty, without hardship, without fear or trembling.

The members of the Fellowship have learned to do this without suffering the loss of any of the joys of living or sacrificing any of their rights as individuals. Nay, they have discovered that the Fellowship way is the only path to enduring happiness.

I have come to tell you about the Fellowship and to place in your hands the MASTER-KEY to all riches.

My identity will not be revealed, for it would be of no benefit to you. If you wish to speak of me you may call me the "Rich Man from Happy Valley."

THE DUAL SELF

Before I describe the Twelve Great Riches let me reveal to you some of the riches you already possess; riches of which most of you may not be conscious.

First, I would have you recognize that each of you is a plural personality, although you may regard yourself as a single personality. You and every other person consist of at least two distinct personalities, and many of you possess more.

There is that self which you recognize when you look into a mirror. That is your physical self. But it is only the house in which your other selves live. In that house there are two individuals at least who are eternally in conflict with each other.

One is a negative sort of person who thinks and moves and lives in an atmosphere of fear and doubt and poverty and ill health. This self expects failure, and seldom is disappointed. It thinks of the circumstances of life which you do not want but which you seem forced to accept—poverty, greed, superstition, fear, doubt, worry and physical sickness.

And one is your "other self," a positive sort of person who thinks in terms of opulence, sound health, love and friendship, personal achievement, creative vision, service to others, and who guides you unerringly to the attainment of all of these blessings. It is this self which alone is capable of recognizing and appropriating the Twelve Great Riches. It is the only self which is capable of receiving the Master-Key to Riches.

These are not imaginary personalities of which I speak. They are real, for they have been revealed through scientific investigation of irreproachable authenticity.

Then you have many other priceless assets of which you may not be aware; hidden riches you have neither recognized nor used. Among these is a modern radio broadcasting and receiving station so powerful that it may pick up and send out the vibrations of thought from or to any part of the world, including the potential capacity to reach out into the cosmos and tune in with the power of Infinite Intelligence.

Your radio station operates automatically and continuously, when you are asleep just as when you are awake.

And it is under the control at all times of one or the other of your two major personalities, the negative personality or the positive personality. When your negative personality is in control your radio station picks up only the negative thought vibrations which are being sent out by hundreds of millions of other negative personalities throughout the world. These are accepted, acted upon and translated into their physical equivalent in terms of the circumstances of life which you do not wish.

When your positive personality is in control it picks up only the positive thought vibrations being released by millions of other positive personalities throughout the world, and translates them into their physical equivalent in terms of prosperity, sound health, love, hope, faith, peace of mind and happiness; the values of life for which you and every other normal person are searching.

I have come to reveal to you the Master-Key by which you may attain these and many other riches. That mysterious key which unlocks the doors to the solution of all human problems, acquires all riches, and places every individual radio station under the control of one's "other self."

I am known as the Rich Man from Happy Valley because I have come into possession of the Master-Key to Riches. The nature of my riches I shall presently reveal to you. But first let me tell you that I was not born to riches.

I was born in poverty and illiteracy.

My formal education has been limited to the knowledge available through a country grade school.

And the entire universe, as far as I was concerned, extended no further than the boundary lines of the backwoods county into which I was born.

Then came a great awakening. Love came into my heart, and with it the influence of the greatest person I shall ever hope to know. She became my wife and guide, for she came from the outer world—that world I had not suspected to exist. She was a woman of culture and education. From her I learned some of the secrets of biology, and chemistry, and astronomy, and physics. She reached deeply into my soul and uncovered that "other self" of which I had no knowledge.

Step by step, patiently and with love, she lifted me into a higher and yet higher plane of understanding, until at long last I was prepared to receive the great Master-Key to Riches—the gift which I shall share with you in the hope that you may become as rich as I.

With that blessing came also a responsibility consisting of an obligation to reveal the secrets of the great Master-Key to as many of you as may prepare yourselves to receive it. But let me here warn you that the Master-Key may be retained only by those who accept the obligation to share it with others. No man may use it selfishly, for his personal aggrandizement alone.

I shall reveal to you the means by which you may share the blessings of the Master-Key, but the responsibility of sharing must become your own.

The founders of the Rotary Club movement must have recognized the benefits of sharing, for they adopted as their motto: *"He profits most who serves best."*

And every close observer must have recognized that all individual successes which endure *have had their beginning through the beneficent influence of some other individual,* through some form of sharing.

My great opportunity consisted in the willingness of my wife to share with me the knowledge which she had acquired, plus the knowledge I gained from the principles which placed the Master-Key within my reach.

Your opportunity may well consist in my willingness to share this knowledge with you. But I have not come to give you material riches alone. I have come to share with you the knowledge by which you may acquire riches—*all riches*—through the expression of *your own personal initiative!*

That is the greatest of all gifts!

And it is the only kind of gift that anyone who is blessed with the advantages of a great nation like ours should expect. For here we have every potential form of riches available to mankind. We have them in great abundance.

So I assume that you too wish to become rich.

Let us become partners in the attainment of your desire, for I have found the way to all riches. Therefore I am prepared to serve as your guide.

I sought the path to riches the hard way before I learned that there is a short and dependable path I could have followed had I been guided as I hope to guide you.

Before we begin our journey to the land of riches let us take inventory so that we may know the true nature of riches. Yes, let us be prepared to recognize riches when we come within their reach.

Some believe that riches consist in money alone!

But enduring riches, in the broader sense, consist in many other values than those of material things, and may I add that without these other intangible values the possession of money will not bring the happiness which some believe it will provide.

When I speak of "riches" I have in mind the greater riches whose possessors have made life pay off on their own terms—the terms of full and complete happiness. I call these the "*Twelve Riches of Life.*" And I sincerely wish to share them with all of you who are prepared to receive them, in whole or in part.

You may wonder about my willingness to share, so I shall tell you that the MASTER-KEY TO RICHES enables its possessors to add to their own store of riches everything of value which they share with others.

This is one of the strangest facts of life, but it is a fact which each of you must recognize and respect if you hope to become as rich as I.

2

DEEDS, CHARACTER AND DESTINY

James Allen

There is, and always has been, a widespread belief in Fate, or Destiny, that is, in an eternal and inscrutable Power which apportions definite ends to both individuals and nations. This belief has arisen from long observation of the facts of life.

Men are conscious that there are certain occurrences which they cannot control, and are powerless to avert. Birth and death, for instance, are inevitable, and many of the incidents of life appear equally inevitable.

Men strain every nerve for the attainment of certain ends, and gradually they become conscious of a Power which seems to be not of themselves, which frustrates their puny efforts, and laughs, as it were, at their fruitless striving and struggle.

As men advance in life, they learn to submit, more or less, to this overruling Power which they do not understand, perceiving only its effects in themselves and the world around them, and they call it by various names, such as God, Providence, Fate, Destiny, etc.

Men of contemplation, such as poets and philosophers, step aside, as it were, to watch the movements of this mysterious Power as it seems to elevate its favorites on the one hand, and strike down its victims on the other, without reference to merit or demerit.

The greatest poets, especially the dramatic poets, represent this Power in their works, as they have observed it in Nature. The Greek and Roman dramatists usually depict their heroes as having foreknowledge of their fate, and taking means to escape it; but by so doing they blindly involve themselves in a series of consequences which bring about the doom which they are trying to avert. Shakespeare's characters, on the other hand, are represented, as in Nature, with no foreknowledge (except in the form of presentiment) of their particular destiny. Thus, according to the poets, whether the man knows his fate or not, he cannot avert it, and every conscious or unconscious act of his is a step towards it.

Omar Khayyam's Moving Finger is a vivid expression of this idea of Fate:

> The Moving Finger writes, and having writ,
> Moves on: nor all thy Piety nor Wit
> Shall lure it back to cancel half a line,
> Nor all thy Tears wash out a Word of it.

Thus, men in all nations and times have experienced in their lives the action of this invincible Power or Law, and in our nation today this experience has been crystallized in the terse proverb, "Man proposes, God disposes."

But, contradictory as it may appear, there is an equally widespread belief in man's responsibility as a free agent.

All moral teaching is an affirmation of man's freedom to choose his course and mold his destiny: and man's patient and untiring efforts in achieving his ends are declarations of consciousness of freedom and power.

This dual experience of fate on the one hand, and freedom

on the other, has given rise to the interminable controversy between the believers in Fatalism and the upholders of free will—a controversy which was recently revived under the term "Determinism versus Free will."

Between apparently conflicting extremes there is always a "middle way" of balance, justice, or compensation which, while it includes both extremes, cannot be said to be either one or the other, and which brings both into harmony; and this middle way is the point of contact between two extremes.

Truth cannot be a partisan, but, by its nature, is the Reconciler of extremes; and so, in the matter which we are considering, there is a "golden mean" which brings Fate and Free will into close relationship, wherein, indeed, it is seen that these two indisputable facts in human life, for such they are, are but two aspects of one central law, one unifying and all-embracing principle, namely, the law of causation in its moral aspect.

Moral causation necessitates both Fate and Free will, both individual responsibility and individual predestination, for the law of causes must also be the law of effects, and cause and effect must always be equal; the train of causation, both in matter and mind, must be eternally balanced, therefore eternally just, eternally perfect. Thus every effect may be said to be a thing preordained, but the predetermining power is a cause, and not the fiat of an arbitrary will.

Man finds himself involved in the train of causation. His life is made up of causes and effects. It is both a sowing and a reaping. Each act of his is a cause which must be balanced by its effects. He chooses the cause (this is Free will), he cannot choose, alter, or avert the effect (this is Fate); thus Free will stands for the power to initiate causes, and destiny is involvement in effects.

It is therefore true that man is predestined to certain ends, but he himself has (though he knows it not) issued the mandate;

that good or evil thing from which there is no escape, he has, by his own deeds, brought about.

It may here be urged that man is not responsible for his deeds, that these are the effects of his character, and that he is not responsible for the character, good or bad, which was given him at his birth. If character was "given him" at birth, this would be true, and there would then be no moral law, and no need for moral teaching; but characters are not given ready made, they are evolved; they are, indeed, effects, the products of the moral law itself, that is—the products of deeds. Character result of an accumulation of deeds which have been piled up, so to speak, by the individual during his life.

Man is the doer of his own deeds; as such he is the maker of his own character; and as the doer of his deeds and the maker of his character, he is the molder and shaper of his destiny. He has the power to modify and alter his deeds, and every time he acts he modifies his character, and with the modification of his character for good or evil, he is predetermining for himself new destinies—destinies disastrous or beneficent in accordance with the nature of his deeds. Character is destiny itself; as a fixed combination of deeds, it bears within itself the results of those deeds. These results lie hidden as moral seeds in the dark recesses of the character, awaiting their season of germination, growth, and fruitage.

Those things which befall a man are the reflections of himself; that destiny which pursued him, which he was powerless to escape by effort, or avert by prayer, was the relentless ghoul of his own wrong deeds demanding and enforcing restitution; those blessings and curses which come to him unbidden are the reverberating echoes of the sounds which he himself sent forth.

It is this knowledge of the Perfect Law working through and above all things; of the Perfect Justice operating in and adjusting all human affairs, that enables the good man to love his enemies, and to rise above all hatred, resentment, and complaining; for he knows that only his own can come to him, and that, though he be surrounded by persecutors, his enemies are but the blind instruments of a faultless retribution; and so he blames them not, but calmly receives his accounts, and patiently pays his moral debts.

But this is not all; he does not merely pay his debts; he takes care not to contract any further debts. He watches himself and makes his deeds faultless. While paying off evil accounts, he is laying up good accounts. By putting an end to his own sin, he is bringing evil and suffering to an end.

And now let us consider how the Law operates in particular instances in the outworking of destiny through deeds and character. First, we will look at this present life, for the present is the synthesis of the entire past; the net result of all that a man has ever thought and done is contained within him. It is noticeable that sometimes the good man fails and the unscrupulous man prospers—a fact which seems to put all moral maxims as to the good results of righteousness out of account—and because of this, many people deny the operation of any just law in human life, and even declare that it is chiefly the unjust that prosper.

Nevertheless, the moral law exists, and is not altered or subverted by shallow conclusions. It should be remembered that man is a changing, evolving being. The good man was not always good; the bad man was not always bad. Even in this life, there was a time, in a large number of instances, when the man who is now just, was unjust; when he who is now kind, was cruel; when he who is now pure, was impure.

Conversely, there was a time in this life, in a number of instances, when he who is now unjust, was just; when he who is now cruel, was kind; when he who is now impure, was pure.

Thus, the good man who is overtaken with calamity today is reaping the result of his former evil sowing; later he will reap the happy result of his present good sowing; while the bad man is now reaping the result of his former good sowing; later he will reap the result of his present sowing of bad.

Characteristics are fixed habits of mind, the results of deeds. An act repeated a large number of times becomes unconscious, or automatic—that is, it then seems to repeat itself without any effort on the part of the doer, so that it seems to him almost impossible not to do it, and then it has become a mental characteristic.

Here is a poor man out of work. He is honest, and is not a shirker. He wants work, and cannot get it. He tries hard, and continues to fail. Where is the justice in his lot? There was a time in this man's condition when he had plenty of work. He felt burdened with it; he shirked it, and longed for ease. He thought how delightful it would be to have nothing to do.

He did not appreciate the blessedness of his lot. His desire for ease is now gratified, but the fruit for which he longed, and which he thought would taste so sweet, has turned to ashes in his mouth. The condition which he aimed for, namely, to have nothing to do, he has reached, and there he is compelled to remain till his lesson is thoroughly learned.

And he is surely learning that habitual ease is degrading, that to have nothing to do is a condition of wretchedness, and that work is a noble and blessed thing. His former desires and deeds have brought him where he is; and now his present desire for work, his ceaseless searching and asking for it, will just as surely bring about its own beneficent result. No longer desiring idleness, his present condition will, as an effect, the cause of which is no longer propagated, soon pass away, and he will obtain employment; and if his whole mind is now set on work, and he desires it above all else, then when it comes he will be overwhelmed with it; it will flow in to him from all sides, and he will prosper in his industry.

Then, if he does not understand the law of cause and effect in human life, he will wonder why work comes to him apparently unsought, while others who seek it strenuously fail to obtain it. Nothing comes unbidden; where the shadow is, there also is the substance. That which comes to the individual is the product of his own deeds.

As cheerful industry leads to greater industry and increasing prosperity, and labor shirked or undertaken discontentedly leads to a lesser degree of labor and decreasing prosperity, so with all the varied conditions of life as we see them—they are the destinies wrought by the thoughts and deeds of each particular individual. So also with the vast variety of characters—they are the ripening and ripened growth of the sowing of deeds.

As the individual reaps what he sows, so the nation, being a community of individuals, reaps also what it sows. Nations become great when their leaders are just men; they fall and fade when their just men pass away. Those who are in power set an example, good or bad, for the entire nation.

Great will be the peace and prosperity of a nation when there shall arise within it a line of statesmen who, having first established themselves in a lofty integrity of character, shall direct the energies of the nation toward the culture of virtue and development of character, knowing that only through personal industry, integrity, and nobility can national prosperity proceed.

Still, above all, is the Great Law, calmly and with infallible justice meting out to mortals their fleeting destinies, tear-stained or smiling, the fabric of their hands. Life is a great school for the development of character, and all, through strife and struggle, vice and virtue, success and failure, are slowly but surely learning the lessons of wisdom.

3

RIGHT BEGINNINGS

James Allen

"All common things, each day's events,
That with the hour begin and end;
Our pleasures and our discontents
Are rounds by which we may ascend."

"We have not wings, we cannot soar;
But we have feet to scale and climb."

—Longfellow

"For common life, its wants
And ways, would I set forth in beauteous hues."

—Browning

Life is full of beginnings. They are presented every day and every hour to every person. Most beginnings are small, and appear trivial and insignificant, but in reality they are the most important things in life.

See how in the material world everything proceeds from small beginnings. The mightiest river is at first a rivulet over which the grasshopper could leap; the great flood commences with a few drops of rain; the sturdy oak, which has endured the storms of a thousand winters, was once an acorn; and the smoldering match, carelessly dropped, may be the means of devastating a whole town by fire.

Consider, also, how in the spiritual world the greatest things proceed from smallest beginnings. A light fancy may be the inception of a wonderful invention or an immortal work of art; a spoken sentence may turn the tide of history; a pure thought entertained may lead to the exercise of a world-wide regenerative power; and a momentary animal impulse may lead to the darkest crime.

Have you yet discovered the vast importance of beginnings? Do you really know what is involved in a beginning? Do you know the number of beginnings you are continuously making, and realise their full import? If not, come with me for a short time, and thoughtfully explore this much ignored byway of blessedness, for blessed it is when wisely resorted to, and much strength and comfort it holds for the understanding mind.

A BEGINNING IS IN ITSELF AN END

A beginning is a cause, and as such it must be followed by an effect, or a train of effects, and the effect will always be of the same nature as the cause. The nature of an initial impulse will always determine the body of its results. A beginning also presupposes an ending, a consummation, achievement, or goal. A gate leads to a path, and the path leads to some particular destination; so a beginning leads to results, and results lead to a completion.

There are right beginnings and wrong beginnings, which are followed by effects of a like nature. You can, by careful thought, avoid wrong beginnings and make right beginnings, and so escape evil results and enjoy good results.

There are beginnings over which you have no control and authority—these are without, in the universe, in the world of nature around you, and in other people who have the same liberty as yourself.

Do not concern yourself with these beginnings, but direct your energies and attention to those beginnings over which you have complete control and authority, and which bring about the complicated web of results which compose your life. These beginnings are to be found in the realm of your own thoughts and actions; in your mental attitude under the variety of circumstances through which you pass; in your conduct day by day—in short, in your life as you make it, which is your world of good or ill.

In aiming at the life of Blessedness one of the simplest beginnings to be considered and rightly made is that which we all make everyday—namely, the beginning of each day's life.

How do you begin each day? At what hour do you rise? How do you commence your duties? In what frame of mind do you enter upon the sacred life of a new day? What answer can you give your heart to these important questions? You will find that much happiness or unhappiness follows upon the right or wrong beginning of the day, and that, when every day is wisely begun, happy and harmonious sequences will mark its course, and life in its totality will not fall far short of the ideal blessedness.

It is a right and strong beginning to the day to rise at an early hour. Even if your worldly duty does not demand it, it is wise to make of it a duty, and begin the day strongly by shaking off indolence. How are you to develop strength of will and mind and body if you begin every day by yielding to weakness? Self-indulgence is always followed by unhappiness. People who lie in bed till a late hour are never bright and cheerful and fresh, but are the prey of irritabilities, depressions, debilities, nervous disorders, abnormal fancies, and all unhappy moods. This is the heavy price which they have to pay for their daily indulgence. Yet, so blinding is the pandering to self that, like the drunkard who takes his daily dram in the belief that it is bracing up the nerves which it is all the time shattering, so the lie-a-bed is convinced that long hours of ease are necessary for him as a possible remedy for those very moods and weaknesses and disorders of which his indulgence is the cause. Men and women are totally unaware of the great losses which they entail by this common indulgence: loss of strength both of mind and body, loss of prosperity, loss of knowledge, and loss of happiness.

Begin the day, then, by rising early. If you have no object in doing so, never mind; get up, and go out for a gentle walk among the beauties of nature, and you will experience a buoyancy, a freshness, and a delight, not to say a peace of mind, which will amply reward you for your effort. One good effort is followed by another; and when a man begins the day by rising early, even though with no other purpose in view, he will find that the silent early hour is conducive to clearness of mind and calmness of thought, and that his early morning walk is enabling him to become a consecutive thinker, and so to see life and its problems, as well as himself and his affairs, in a clearer light; and so in time he will rise early with the express purpose of preparing and harmonising his mind to meet any and every difficulty with wisdom and calm strength.

There is, indeed, a spiritual influence in the early morning hour, a divine silence and an inexpressible repose, and he who, purposeful and strong, throws off the mantle of ease and climbs the hills to greet the morning sun will thereby climb no inconsiderable distance up the hills of blessedness and truth.

The right beginning of the day will be followed by

cheerfulness at the morning meal, permeating the house-hold with a sunny influence; and the tasks and duties of the day will be undertaken in a strong and confident spirit, and the whole day will be well lived.

Then there is a sense in which every day may be regarded as the beginning of a new life, in which one can think, act, and live newly, and in a wiser and better spirit.

> Every day is a fresh beginning;
> Every morn is the world made new,
> Ye who are weary of sorrow and sinning,
> Here is a beautiful hope for you,
> A hope for me and a hope for you.

THOUGHTS AS BUILDING BLOCKS

Do not dwell upon the sins and mistakes of yesterday so exclusively as to have no energy and mind left for living rightly today, and do not think that the sins of yesterday can prevent you from living purely today. Begin today aright, and, aided by the accumulated experiences of all your past days, live it better than any of your previous days; but you cannot possibly live it better unless you begin it better. The character of the whole day depends upon the way it is begun.

Another beginning which is of great importance is the beginning of any particular and responsible undertaking. How does a man begin the building of a house? He first secures a plan of the proposed edifice and then proceeds to build according to the plan, scrupulously following it in every detail, beginning with the foundation. Should he neglect the beginning—namely, the obtaining of a mathematical plan—his labor would be wasted, and his building, should it reach completion without tumbling to pieces, would be insecure and worthless. The same law holds good in any important work: the right beginning and first essential is *a definite mental plan on which to build*. Nature will have no slipshod work, no slovenliness, and she annihilates confusion, or rather, confusion is in itself annihilation. Order, definiteness, purpose eternally and universally prevail, and he who in his operations ignores these mathematical elements at once deprives himself of substantiality, completeness, success.

> Life without a plan,
> As useless as the moment it began,
> Serves merely as a soil for discontent
> To thrive in, an encumbrance ere half spent.

Let a man start in business without having in his mind a perfectly formed plan to systematically pursue and he will be incoherent in his efforts and will fail in his business operations. The laws which must be observed in the building of a house also operate in the building up of a business. A definite plan is followed by coherent effort; and coherent effort is followed by well-knit and orderly results—to wit, completeness, perfection, success, happiness.

But not only mechanical and commercial enterprise— all undertakings, of whatsoever nature, come under this law. The author's book, the artist's picture, the orator's speech, the reformer's work, the inventor's machine, the general's campaign, are all carefully planned in the mind before the attempt to actualise them is commenced; and in accordance with the unity, solidarity, and perfection of the original mental plan will be the actual and ultimate success of the undertaking.

Successful men, influential men, good men are those who, amongst other things, have learned the value and utilised the power which lies hidden in those obscure beginnings which the foolish man passes by as "insignificant."

But the most important beginning of all—that upon which afflication or blessedness inevitably depends, yet is most neglected and least understood—is the inception of thought in the hidden, but causal region of the mind. Your whole life is a series of effects having their cause in thought—in your own thought. All conduct is made and moulded by thought; all deeds, good or bad, are thoughts made visible. A seed put into the ground is the beginning of a plant or tree; the seed germinates, the plant or tree comes forth into the light and evolves. A thought put into the mind is the beginning of a line of conduct: the thought first sends down its roots into the mind, and then pushes forth into the light in the forms of actions or conduct, which evolve into character and destiny.

Hateful, angry, envious, covetous, and impure thoughts are wrong beginnings, which lead to painful results. Loving, gentle, kind, unselfish and pure thoughts are right beginnings, which lead to blissful results. This is so simple, so plain, so absolutely true! and yet how neglected, how evaded, and how little understood!

The gardener who most carefully studies how, when, and where to put in his seeds obtains the best results and gains the greater horticultural knowledge. The best crops gladden the soul of him who makes the best beginning. The man who most patiently studies how to put into his mind the seeds of strong, wholesome, and charitable thoughts, will obtain the best results in life, and will gain greater knowledge of truth. The greatest blessedness comes to him, who infuses into his mind the purest and noblest thoughts.

None but right acts can follow right thoughts; none but a right life can follow right acts—and by living a right life all blessedness is achieved.

He who considers the nature and import of his thoughts, who strives daily to eliminate bad thoughts and supplant them with good, comes at last to see that thoughts are the beginnings of results which affect every fibre of his being, which potently influence every event and circumstance of his life. And when he thus sees, he thinks only right thoughts, chooses to make only those mental beginnings which lead to peace and blessedness.

Wrong thoughts are painful in their inception, painful in their growth, and painful in their fruitage. Right thoughts are blissful in their inception, blissful in their growth, and blissful in their fruitage.

Many are the right beginnings which a man must discover and adopt on his way to wisdom; but that which is first and last, most important and all embracing, which is the source and fountain of all abiding happiness, is the right beginning of the mental operations—this implies the steady development of self-control, will-power, steadfastness, strength, purity, gentleness, insight, and comprehension. It leads to the perfecting of life, for he who thinks perfectly has abolished all unhappiness, his every moment is peaceful, his years are rounded with bliss—he has attained to the complete and perfect blessedness.

4

THE 17 PRINCIPLES OF SUCCESS

Napoleon Hill

A FAST REVIEW

The list that follows is meant to serve as a reminder. Look it over once a week. Are you making regular progress in each of these areas? If you routinely evaluate your efforts to embrace the principles, you are less likely to be caught in a crisis because you've neglected to think accurately, for instance, or to find that your coworkers suddenly regard you as an opportunistic shark.

1. Develop definiteness of purpose.
2. Establish a mastermind alliance.
3. Assemble an attractive personality.
4. Use applied faith.
5. Go the extra mile.
6. reate personal initiative.
7. Build a positive mental attitude.
8. Control your enthusiasm.
9. Enforce self-discipline
10. Think accurately.
11. Control your attention.
12. Inspire teamwork.

13. Learn from adversity and defeat.
14. Cultivate creative vision.
15. Maintain sound health.
16. Budget your time and money.
17. Use cosmic habitforce,

A DETAILED EVALUATION

Following are concise summaries of the steps to making each principle a part of your life. Read them through and then use the lines provided at the end of each section to write down specific actions you plan to take to implement the principles.

The summaries themselves will give you concrete recommendations about what to do. Under the definiteness of purpose you might write down that you will define your major goal, write out a plan for achieving it, and read that plan aloud to yourself every day, all of which are mentioned in the summary. But if you also include a date by which you will have your plan written down, you will be making a commitment to yourself that will provide you with extra motivation. So do not simply parrot back the summary's suggestions; consider carefully the changes you need to make and be as detailed as possible in writing them out. In a few weeks or months you can look at these notes, recognize the progress you've made, and renew your commitment to success.

1. DEVELOP DEFINITENESS OF PURPOSE—WITH PMA

The Starting Point of All Worthwhile Achievements

You should have one high, desirable, outstanding goal, and keep it ever before you. You can have many nonconflicting goals which help you to reach your major definite goal. It is advisable to have immediate, intermediate, and distant objectives. When you set a definite major goal, you are apt to recognize that which will help you achieve it.

Determine or fix in your mind exactly what you desire. Be definite.

Evaluate and determine exactly what you will give in return.

Set a definite date for exactly when you intend to possess your desire.

Identify your desire with a definite plan for carrying out and achieving your objective. Put your plan into action at once.

Clearly define your plan for achievement. Write out precisely and concisely exactly what you want, exactly when you want to achieve it, and exactly what you intend to give in return.

Each and every day, morning and evening, read your written statement aloud. As you read it, see, feel, and believe yourself already in possession of your objective.

Engage in personal inspection with regularity to determine whether you are on the right track and headed in the right direction so that you don't deviate from the path that leads to the achievement of your objective.

To guarantee success, engage daily in study, thinking, and planning time with PMA regarding yourself and your family and how you can achieve your definite goals.

WHATEVER YOUR MIND CAN CONCEIVE AND BELIEVE, YOU CAN ACHIEVE—WHEN YOU HAVE PMA AND APPLY IT.

2. ESTABLISH A MASTERMIND ALLIANCE—WITH PMA

A mastermind alliance is two or more minds working together in the spirit of perfect harmony toward the attainment of a specific objective.

This principle makes it possible for you, through association with others, to acquire and utilize the knowledge and experience needed for the attainment of any desired goal in

Your mastermind alliance can be created by surrounding yourself or aligning yourself with the advice, counsel, and personal cooperation of several people who are willing to lend you their wholehearted aid for the attainment of your objective in the spirit of perfect harmony.

You can create a mastermind alliance with your spouse, your manager, a friend, a coworker, etc. Once a mastermind alliance is formed, the group as a whole must become and remain active. The group must move in a definite plan, at a definite time, toward a definite common objective. Indecision, inactivity, or delay will destroy usefulness of the alliance. There must be a complete meeting of the minds without reservations on the part of any member.

You can have several mastermind alliances, each with different objectives—i.e., an alliance with your spouse to reach your family objectives, an alliance with your banker or investment counselor or attorney for your financial objectives, an alliance with your minister or clergy for your spiritual objectives, etc.

3. ASSEMBLE AN ATTRACTIVE PERSONALITY—WITH PMA

Your personality is your greatest asset or greatest liability, for it embraces everything that you control: mind, body, and soul. A person's personality is the person. It shapes the nature of your thoughts, your deeds, your relationships with others, and it establishes the boundaries of the space you occupy in the world.

It is essential that you develop a pleasing personality—pleasing to yourself and to others.

It is imperative that you develop the habit of being sensitive to your own reactions to individuals, circumstances, and events and to the reactions of individuals and groups to what you say, think, or do.

Positive Factors of a Pleasing Personality

- A positive mental attitude
- Tolerance
- Alertness
- Common courtesy
- A fondness for people
- Flexibility
- Tactfulness
- Personal magnetism
- A pleasant tone of voice
- Control of facial expressions
- Sportsmanship
- Sincerity
- A sense of humor
- Humility of the heart
- Smiling
- Enthusiasm Control of temper and emotions
- Patience
- Proper dress

DO UNTO OTHERS AS YOU WOULD HAVE OTHERS DO UNTO YOU.

4. USE APPLIED FAITH—WITH PMA

Faith is a state of mind through which your aims, desires, plans, and purposes may be translated into their physical or financial equivalent.

Applied faith means action—specifically, the habit of applying your faith under any and all circumstances. It is faith in your God, yourself, your fellowman—and the unlimited opportunities available to you.

Faith without action is dead. Faith is the art of believing by doing. It comes as a result of persistent action. Fear and doubt are faith in reverse gear. Faith, in its positive application, is the key which will give one direct communications with Infinite Intelligence.

Applied faith is belief in an objective or purpose backed by unqualified activity. If you want results, try a prayer. When you pray, express your gratitude, and thanksgiving for the blessings you already have received; then ask the Good Lord for his help. Affirm the objectives of your desires through prayer each night and morning. Inspire your imagination to see yourself already in possession of them, and act precisely as if you were already in physical possession of them. The possession of anything first takes place mentally by being imagined in the mind's eye.

PRAYER IS YOUR GREATEST POWER!

5. GO THE EXTRA MILE—WITH PMA

Render more and better service for which you are paid, and do it with a positive mental attitude. Form the habit of going the extra mile because of the pleasure you get out of it and because of what it does to you and for you deep down inside. It is inevitable that every seed of useful service you sow will multiply itself and come back to you in overwhelming abundance.

Following this principle will make you indispensable to other people. The principle manifests itself in two important laws: the Law of Compensation and the Law of Increasing Returns. These unvarying laws always reward intelligent effort rendered in the attitude of faith and rendered instinctively without regards to the limits of immediate compensation.

The quality of the service rendered plus the quantity of the service rendered plus the mental attitude in which it is rendered equals your compensation in the world and the amount of space you will occupy in the hearts of your fellow man.

MAKE GOING THE EXTRA MILE WITH PMA A HABIT!

6. CREATE PERSONAL INITIATIVE—WITH PMA

Personal initiative is the inner power that starts all action. It is the power that inspires the completion of that which one begins. It is the dynamo that starts the faculty of the imagination into action.

It is, in fact, Self-motivation.

Motivation is that which induces action or determines choice. It is that which provides a motive. A motive is that inner urge only within the individual which incites you to action, such as an idea, an emotion, a desire, or an impulse. It is a hope or other force which starts in an attempt to produce specific results.

When you know principles that can motivate you, you will then know principles that can motivate others.

Motivate yourself with PMA. Hope is the magic ingredient in motivation, but the secret of accomplishment is getting into action.

USE AND DEVELOP THE SELF-STARTER. DO IT NOW!

7. BUILD A POSITIVE MENTAL ATTITUDE

PMA stands for "positive mental attitude."

A positive mental attitude is the right, honest, constructive thought, action, or reaction to any person, situation, or set of circumstances that does not violate the laws of God or the right of one's fellowman.

PMA allows you to build on hope and overcome the negative attitudes of despair and discouragement. It gives you the mental power, the feeling, the confidence to do anything you make up your mind to do. PMA is commonly referred to as the "I can…I will" attitude applicable to all challenging circumstances in your life.

You create and maintain a positive mental attitude through your own willpower, based on motives of your own adaption. To develop PMA, strive to understand and apply the Golden Rule; be considerate and sensitive to the reactions of others; be sensitive to your own reactions by controlling your emotional responses; be a good finder; believe that any goal can be achieved; and develop what are understood to be right habits of thought and action.

A positive mental attitude is the catalyst necessary for achieving worthwhile success. Achievement is attained through some combination of PMA and definiteness of purpose with one or more of the other fifteen success principles.

MAINTAIN THE RIGHT ATTITUDE—A POSITIVE MENTAL ATTITUDE.

8. CONTROL YOUR ENTHUSIASM—WITH PMA

A person without enthusiasm is like a watch without a mainspring. Father John O'Brien, research professor of theology at the University of Notre Dame, says, "the first ingredient which I believe is absolutely necessary for a successful, efficient, and competent individual is enthusiasm." He adds, "Enthusiasm comes from the Greek words that let you look into the root of this word—into its basic, fundamental and original meaning. The first is *theos*, which means God. The other two words are *en-Tae*, so that in the early usage of this term of the ancient Greeks, it literally meant, 'God within you.'" Further: "No battle of any importance can be won without enthusiasm."

To become enthusiastic about achieving a desirable goal, keep your mind on that goal day after day. The more worthy and desirable your objectives, the more dedicated and enthusiastic you will become. Understand and act on William James's statement: "The emotions are not always immediately subject to reason but they are always immediately subject to ACTION" (emphasis added). Enthusiasm thrives on a positive mind and positive action. This is the key to controlling your enthusiasm: always give it a worthy goal to focus on and once you have channeled it toward that goal, it will carry you forward.

Real enthusiasm comes from within. However, enthusiasm is like getting water from a well; first you have to prime the pump but soon the water flows and flows and flows. You can be enthusiastic about everything and anything you know or do. Enthusiasm is a PMA characteristic. It can be generated naturally from one's thoughts, feelings and emotions, but more important, it can be generated at will.

TO BE ENTHUSIASTIC… ACT ENTHUSIASTICALLY!

9. ENFORCE SELF-DISCIPLINE—WITH PMA

Self-discipline enables you to develop control over yourself. Self-discipline begins with mastery of your thoughts, what you really are, what you really do. Your failures and your successes are the results of habits. We are creatures of habit, but because we are minds with bodies, we can change our habits.

Self-discipline is perhaps the most important function in aiding an individual in the development and maintenance of habits of thought which enable that person to fix his or her entire attention upon any desired purpose and to hold it there until that purpose has been attained.

If you do not control your thoughts, you do not control your deeds. Think first and act afterward. Self-discipline is the principle by which you may voluntarily shape the patterns of your thoughts to harmonize with your goals and purposes.

DIRECT YOUR THOUGHTS, CONTROL YOUR EMOTIONS, ORDAIN YOUR DESTINY WITH PMA.

10. THINK ACCURATELY—WITH PMA

Accurate thinking is based on two major fundamentals:

1. Inductive reasoning, based on the assumption of unknown facts or hypotheses.
2. Deductive reasoning, based on known facts or what are believed to be facts.

In school we are taught deductive and inductive reasoning and the fallacy that results in starting with the wrong premise in the one instance and making the wrong inference in the other. Accurate thinking and common sense are in part the result of experiences. You can learn from your own experiences as well as those of others when you learn how to recognize, relate, assimilate, and apply principles in order to achieve your goals.

1. Separate facts from fiction or hearsay evidence.
2. Separate facts into classes: important and unimportant.

Be careful of others' opinions. They could be dangerous and destructive. Make sure your opinions are not someone else's prejudices. The accurate thinker learns to use his or her own judgment and to be cautious no matter who may endeavor to influence him or her.

TRUTH WILL BE TRUTH REGARDLESS OF A CLOSED MIND, IGNORANCE, OR REFUSAL TO BELIEVE.

11. CONTROL YOUR ATTENTION—WITH PMA

Controlled attention is organized mind power. It is the highest form of self-discipline. Controlled attention is the act of coordinating all the faculties of the mind and directing their combined power to a given end or definite objective. It is an act that can be obtained only by the strictest sort of self-discipline.

It is obvious, therefore, that when you voluntarily fix your attention upon a definite major purpose of a positive nature and force your mind through your daily habits of thought to dwell on the subject, you condition your subconscious mind to act on that purpose. Controlled attention, when it is focused upon the object of your definite major purpose, is a medium by which you make positive application of the principle of suggestion.

The mind never remains inactive, not even during sleep. It works continuously by reactions to the influences which reach it. Therefore, the object of controlled attention is that of keeping your mind busy with thought material which may be helpful in attaining the object of your desire.

Controlled attention is self-mastery of the highest order, for it is an accepted fact that the person who controls his or her own mind may control everything else.

KEEP YOUR MIND ON THE THINGS YOU WANT AND OFF THE THINGS YOU DON'T WANT.

12. INSPIRE TEAMWORK—WITH PMA

Teamwork is a willing cooperation and the coordination of effort to achieve a specific objective. When the spirit of teamwork is willing, voluntary, and free, it leads to the attainment of great and enduring power.

It is a system which coordinates all the team players' resources and talents and automatically discourages dishonesty and unfairness, while it adequately compensates the individuals who serve honestly and unselfishly.

The principle of teamwork differs from the mastermind principle in that it is based on the coordination of effort without necessarily embracing the principle of definiteness of purpose or the principle of harmony, two important essentials of the mastermind.

Teamwork produces power, but the question of whether the power is temporary or permanent depends on the motive that inspired the cooperation. If the motive is one that inspires people to cooperate willingly, the power produced by this sort of teamwork will endure as long as that spirit of willingness prevails.

Teamwork builds individuals and businesses and provides unlimited opportunity for all. It is sharing a part of what you have—a part that is good—with others.

THAT WHICH YOU SHARE WILL MULTIPLY; THAT

WHICH YOU WITHHOLD WILL DIMINISH.

13. LEARN FROM ADVERSITY AND DEFEAT—WITH PMA

Every adversity carries with it the seed of an equivalent or greater benefit for those who have PMA and apply it.

Defeat may be a stepping-stone or a stumbling block, according to your mental attitude and how you relate it to yourself.

It is never the same as failure unless and until it has been accepted as such.

Your mental attitude in respect to defeat is the factor of major importance which determines whether you ride with tides of fortune or misfortune. The person with a positive metal attitude reacts to defeat in the spirit of determinaion not to accept it. The person with a negative mental attitude reacts to defeat in the spirit of hopeless acceptance.

THE WORST THING THAT HAPPENS TO YOU MAY BE THE BEST THING THAT CAN HAPPEN TO YOU IF YOU DON'T LET IT GET THE BEST OF YOU.

14. CULTIVATE CREATIVE VISION—WITH PMA

Man's greatest gift is his thinking mind. It analyzes, compares, chooses. It creates, visualizes, foresees, and generates ideas.

Imagination is your mind's exercise, challenge, and adventure. It is the key to all of a person's achievements, the mainspring of all human endeavor, the secret door to the soul of a person. Imagination inspires human endeavor in connection with material things and ideas associated with material things.

Imagination is the workshop of the human mind, where

old ideas and established facts may be assembled into new combinations and put to new uses. It is the act of constructive intellect in the grouping of materials, knowledge, or thoughts into new, original, and rational systems, a constructive or creative faculty embracing poetic, artistic, philosophical, scientific, and ethical imagination.

Creative vision may be an inborn quality of the mind or an acquired quality, for it may be developed by the free and fearless use of the faculty of imagination.

Creative vision extends beyond interest in material things. It judges the future by the past and concerns itself with the future more than with the past. Imagination is influenced and controlled by the powers of reason and experience. Creative vision pushes these aside and attains its ends by basically new ideas and methods.

One of the ways to increase your flow of ideas is by developing the habit of taking study time, thinking time, and planning time. Be quiet and motionless, and listen for that small, still voice that speaks from within as you contemplate the ways in which you can achieve your objectives.

WHAT CAN BE CONCEIVED CAN BE CREATED—WITH PMA.

15. MAINTAIN SOUND HEALTH—WITH PMA

You are a mind with a body. Inasmuch as your brain controls your body, recognize that sound physical health demands a positive mental attitude, a health consciousness. Establish good, well-balanced health habits in work, play, rest, nourishment, and study. To maintain a health consciousness, think in terms of good physical health, not in terms of illness or disease. Remember, what your mind focuses upon, your mind brings into existence, whether it is financial success or physical health.

To maintain a positive attitude for the development and maintenance of a sound health consciousness, use self-discipline, keep your mind free of negative thoughts and influence, and create and maintain a well-balanced life. Follow work with play, mental effort with physical effort, seriousness with humor, and you will be on the road to good health and happiness.

A sound mind and a sound body are attainable if you will put PMA to work for you. Remember, you can enjoy good health and live longer with PMA.

I FEEL HEALTHY! I FEEL HAPPY! I FEEL TERRIFIC!

16. BUDGET YOUR TIME AND MONEY—WITH PMA

Intelligently balance your use of time and resources, both business and personal. Take inventory of yourself and your activities so that you discover where and how you are spending your time and your money.

Engage in study, thinking, and planning time.

Don't waste your time or your money. Ten percent of all you earn is yours to keep and invest. Like any good business, budget your money. Use your time wisely toward attainment of your objectives. Develop a plan for the use of your income for expenses, savings, and investments.

YOU DON'T ALWAYS GET WHAT YOU EXPECT UNLESS YOU INSPECT—WITH PMA.

17. USE COSMIC HABITFORCE—WITH PMA

Cosmic habitforce pertains to the entire universe and is the law by which the equilibrium of the universe is maintained through established patterns or habits. It is the law which forces every living creature and every particle of matter to come under the dominating influence of its environment, including the physical habits and thought habits of humankind.

Cosmic habitforces are the powers which you apply with PMA when you use the universal laws or principles. Cosmic habitforces are employed when you use your mind powers whether they pertain to your conscious or subconscious mind. That is how you think and grow richer or achieve anything in life you desire (in principle) that doesn't violate the laws of God or the rights of your fellowman.

All of us are ruled by habits. These are fastened upon us by repeated thoughts and experiences. You have complete right of control over your thoughts. We create patterns of thought by repeating certain ideas or behavior until the Law of Cosmic Habitforce takes over those patterns and makes them more or less permanent unless or until you consciously rearrange them.

Habits: You have them—some good, perhaps others bad. Many you are aware of, but some that are undesirable you are blinded to. Each begins in your mind consciously or subconsciously. And each can be developed and neutralized or changed at will through the proper use of your mind. You have this power.

You are ruled by your habits. It takes a habit to replace a habit. Develop positive habits that will be in harmony with the achievement of your definite purpose or goal.

SOW AN ACT, AND YOU REAP A HABIT.
SOW A HABIT, AND YOU REAP A CHARACTER.
SOW A CHARACTER, AND YOU REAP A DESTINY.

5

INITIATIVE AND LEADERSHIP

Napoleon Hill

WHEN YOU DO NOT KNOW WHAT TO DO OR WHICH WAY TO TURN, smile. This will relax your mind and let the sunshine of HAPPINESS INTO YOUR SOUL.

"YOU CAN DO IT IF YOU BELIEVE YOU CAN!"

Before you proceed to the mastery of this lesson your attention is directed to the fact that there is perfect co-ordination of thought running throughout this course. You will observe that the entire sixteen lessons harmonize and blend with each other so that they constitute a perfect chain that has been built, link by link, out of the factors that enter into the development of power through organized effort.

You will observe, also, that the same fundamental principles of Applied Psychology form the foundation of each of these lessons, although different application is made of these principles in each of the lessons.

This lesson, on Initiative and leadership, follows the lesson on Self-confidence for the reason that no one could become an efficient leader or take the initiative in any great undertaking without belief in himself.

Initiative and Leadership are associated terms in this lesson for the reason that leadership is essential for the attainment of Success, and Initiative is the very foundation upon which this necessary quality of leadership is built. Initiative is as essential to success as a hub is essential to a wagon wheel.

And what is Initiative?

It is that exceedingly rare quality that prompts—nay, impels—a person to do that which ought to be done without being told to do it. Elbert Hubbard expressed himself on the subject of initiative in the words:

"The world bestows its big prizes, both in money and honors, for one thing, and that is Initiative.

"What is initiative? I'll tell you: It is doing the right thing without being told.

"But next to doing the right thing without being told is to do it when you are told once. That is say, 'Carry the message to Garcia.' Those who can carry a message get high honors, but their pay is not always in proportion.

"Next, there are those who do the right thing when necessity kicks them from behind, and these get indifference instead of honors, and a pittance for pay.

"This kind spend most of the time polishing a bench with a hard luck story.

"Then, still lower down in the scale than this we have the fellow who will not do the right thing even when someone goes along to show him how and stays to see that he does it; he is always out of a job, a receives the contempt he deserves, unless he has a rich pa, in which case destiny patiently waits around the comer with a stuffed club.

"To which class do you belong?"

Inasmuch as you will be expected to take inventory of yourself and determine which of the fifteen factors of this course you need most, after you have completed the sixteenth lesson, it may be well if you begin to get ready for this analysis by answering the question that Elbert Hubbard has asked:

To which class do you belong?

One of the peculiarities of Leadership is the fact that it is never found in those who have not acquired the habit of taking the initiative. Leadership is something that you must invite yourself into; it will never thrust itself upon you. If you will carefully analyze all leaders whom you know you will see that they not only exercised Initiative, but they went about their work with a definite purpose in mind. You will also see that they possessed that quality described in the third lesson of this course, Self-confidence.

These facts are mentioned in this lesson for the reason that it will profit you to observe that successful people make use of all the factors covered by the sixteen lessons of the course; and, for the more important reason that it will profit you to understand thoroughly the principle of organized effort which this Reading Course is intended to establish in your mind.

This seems an appropriate place to state that this course is not intended as a shortcut to success, nor is it intended as a mechanical formula that you may use in noteworthy achievement without effort on your part. The real value of the course lies in the use that you will make of it, and not in the course itself. The chief purpose of the course is to help you develop in yourself the fifteen qualities covered by the sixteen lessons of the course, and one of the most important of these qualities is Initiative, the subject of this lesson.

We will now proceed to apply the principle upon which this lesson is founded by describing, in detail, just how it served successfully to complete a business transaction which most people would call difficult.

In 1916 I needed $25,000.00 with which to create an educational institution, but I had neither this sum nor sufficient collateral with which to borrow it through the usual banking sources. Did I bemoan my fate or think of what I might accomplish if some rich relative or Good Samaritan would come to my rescue by loaning me the necessary capital?

I did nothing of the sort!

I did just what you will be advised, throughout this course, to do. First of all, I made the securing of this capital my definite chief aim. Second, I laid out a complete plan through which to transform this aim into reality. Backed by sufficient Self-confidence and spurred on by Initiative, I proceeded to put my plan into action. But, before the "action" stage of the plan had been reached, more than six weeks of constant, persistent study and effort and thought were embodied in it. If a plan is to be sound it must be built of carefully chosen material.

You will here observe the application of the principle of organized effort, through the operation of which it is possible for one to ally or associate several interests in such a way that each of these interests is greatly strengthened and each supports all the others, just as one link in a chain supports all the other links.

I wanted this $25,000.00 in capital for the purpose of creating a school of Advertising and Salesmanship. Two things were necessary for the organization of such a school. One was the $25,000.00 capital, which I did not have, and the other was the proper course of instruction, which I did have. My problem was to ally myself with some group of men who needed that which I had, and who would supply the $25,000.00. This alliance had to be made through a plan that would benefit all concerned.

After my plan had been completed, and I was satisfied that it was equitable and sound, I laid it before the owner of a well known and reputable business college which just then was finding competition quite keen and was badly in need of a plan for meeting this competition.

My plan was presented in about these words:

Whereas, you have one of the most reputable business colleges in the city; and,

Whereas, you need some plan with which to meet the stiff competition in your field; and,

Whereas, your good reputation has provided you with all the credit you need; and,

Whereas, I have the plan that will help you meet this competition successfully.

Be it resolved, that we ally ourselves through a plan that will give you that which you need and at the same time supply me with something which I need.

Then I proceeded to unfold my plan, further, in these words:

I have written a very practical course on Advertising and Salesmanship. Having built this course out of my actual experience in training and directing salesmen and my experience in planning and Directing many successful advertising campaigns, I have back of it plenty of evidence of its soundness.

If you will use your credit in helping market this course I will place it in your business college, as one of the regular departments of your curriculum and take entire charge of this newly created department. No other business college in the city will be able to meet your competition, for the reason that no other college has such a course as this. The advertising that you do in marketing this course will serve, also, to stimulate the demand for your regular business course. You may charge the entire amount that you spend for this advertising, to my department, and the advertising bill will be paid out of that department, leaving you the accumulative advantage that will accrue to your other departments without cost to you.

Now, I suppose you will want to know where I profit by this transaction, and I will tell you. I want you to enter into a contract with me in which it will be agreed that when the cash receipts from my department equal the amount that you have paid out or contracted to pay out for advertising, my department and my course in Advertising and Salesmanship become my own and I may have the privilege of separating this department from your school and running it under my own name.

The plan was agreeable and the contract was closed.

(Please keep in mind that my definite purpose was to secure the use of $25,000.00 for which I had no security to offer.)

In a little less than a year the Business College had paid out slightly more than $25,000.00 for advertising and marketing my course and the other expenses incidental to the operation of this newly organized department, while the department had collected and, turned back to the College, in tuition fees, a sum equaling the amount the College had spent, and I took the department over, as a going and self-sustaining business, according to the terms of my contract.

As a matter of fact this newly created department not only served to attract students for the other departments of the College, but at the same time the tuition fees collected through this new department were sufficient to place it on a self-sustaining basis before the end of the first year.

Now you can see that while the College did not loan me one penny of actual capital, it nevertheless supplied me with credit which served exactly the same purpose.

I said that my plan was founded upon equity; that it contemplated a benefit to all parties concerned. The benefit accruing to me was the use of the $25,000.00, which resulted in an established and self-sustaining business by the end of the first year. The benefit accruing to the college was the students secured for its regular commercial and business course as a result of the money spent in advertising my department, all advertising having been done under the name of the College.

Today that business college is one of the most successful schools of its kind, and it stands as a monument of sound evidence with which to demonstrate the value of allied effort.

This incident has been related, not alone because it shows the value of initiative and leadership, but for the reason that it leads up to the subject covered by the next lesson of this Reading Course on the Law of Success, which is imagination.

There are generally many plans through the operation of which a desired object may be achieved, and it often happens to be true that the obvious and usual methods employed are not the best. The usual method of procedure, in the case related, would have been that of borrowing from a bank. You can see that this method was impractical, in this case, for the reason that no collateral was available.

A great philosopher once said: "Initiative is the pass-key that opens the door to opportunity."

I do not recall who this philosopher was, but I know that he was great because of the soundness of his statement.

We will now proceed to outline the exact procedure that

you must follow if you are to become a person of initiative and leadership.

First: You must master the habit of procrastination and eliminate it from your make-up. This habit of putting off until tomorrow that which you should have done last week or last year or a score of years ago is gnawing at the very vitals of your being, and you can accomplish nothing until you throw it off.

The method through which you eliminate procrastination is based upon a well known and scientifically tested principle of psychology which has been referred to in the two preceding lessons of this course as Auto-suggestion.

Copy the following formula and place it conspicuously in your room where you will see it as you retire at night and as you arise in the morning:

INITIATIVE AND LEADERSHIP

Having chosen a definite chief aim as my lifework I now understand it to be my duty to transform this purpose into reality.

Therefore, I will form the habit of taking some definite action each day that will carry me one step nearer the attainment of my definite chief aim.

I know that procrastination is a deadly enemy of all who would become leaders in any undertaking, and I will eliminate this habit from my make-up by:

(a) Doing some one definite thing each day, that ought to be done, without anyone telling me to do it.

(b) Looking around until I find at least one thing that I can do each day, that I have not been in the habit of doing, and that will be of value to others, without expectation of pay.

(c) Telling at least one other person, each day, of the

value of practicing this habit of doing something that ought to be done without being told to do it.

I can see that the muscles of the body become strong in proportion to the extent to which they are used, therefore I understand that the habit of initiative also becomes fixed in proportion to the extent that it is practiced.

I realize that the place to begin developing the habit of initiative is in the small, commonplace things connected with my daily work, therefore I will go at my work each day as if I were doing it solely for the purpose of developing this necessary habit of initiative.

I understand that by practicing this habit of taking the initiative in connection with my daily work I will be not only developing that habit, but I will also be attracting the attention of those who will place greater value on my services as a result of this practice.

Signed...

Regardless of what you are now doing, every day brings you face to face with a chance to render some service, outside of the course of your regular duties, that will be of value to others. In rendering this additional service, of your own accord, you of course understand that you are not doing so with the object of receiving monetary pay. You are rendering this service because it provides you with ways and means of exercising, developing and making stronger the aggressive spirit of initiative which you must possess before you can ever become an outstanding figure in the affairs of your chosen field of life-work.

Those who work for money alone, and who receive for their pay nothing but money, are always underpaid, no matter how much they receive. Money is necessary, but the big prizes of life cannot be measured in dollars and cents.

No amount of money could possibly be made to take the place of the happiness and joy and pride that belong to the person who digs a better ditch, or builds a better chicken coop, or sweeps a cleaner floor, or cooks a better meal. Every normal person loves to create something that is better than the average. The joy of creating a work of art is a joy that cannot be replaced by money or any other form of material possession.

I have in my employ a young lady who opens, assorts and answers much of my personal mail. She began in my employ more than three years ago. Then her duties were to take dictation when she was asked to do so. Her salary was about the same as that which others receive for similar service. One day I dictated the following motto which I asked her to typewrite tor me:

Remember that your only limitation is the one that you set up in your own mind.

As she handed the typewritten page back to me she said, "Your motto has given me an idea that is going to be of value to both you and me."

I told her I was glad to have been of service to her. The incident made no particular impression on my mind, but from that day on I could see that it had made a tremendous impression on her mind. She began to come back to the office after supper and performed service that she was neither paid for nor expected to perform. Without anyone telling her to do it she began to bring to my desk letters that she had answered for me. She had studied my style and these letters were attended to as well as I could have done it; in some instances much better. She kept up this habit until my personal secretary resigned. When I began to look for someone to take his place, what was more natural than to turn to this young woman to fill the place. Before I had time to give her the position she took it on her initiative. My personal mail began to come to my desk with a new secretary's name attached, and she was that secretary. On her own time, after hours, without additional pay, she had prepared herself for the best position on my staff.

But that is not all. This young lady became so noticeably efficient that she began to attract the attention of others who offered her attractive positions. I have increased her salary many times and she now receives a salary more than four times as large as the amount she received when she first went to work for me as an ordinary stenographer, and, to tell you the truth, I am helpless in the matter, because she has made herself so valuable to me that I cannot get along without her.

That is initiative transformed into practical, understandable terms. I would be remiss in my duties if I failed to direct your attention to an advantage, other than a greatly increased salary, that this young lady's initiative has brought her. It has developed in her a spirit of cheerfulness that brings her happiness which most stenographers never know. Her work is not work—it is a great interesting game at which she is playing. Even though she arrives at the office ahead of the regular stenographers and remains there long after they have watched the clock tick off five o'clock and quitting time, her hours are shorter by far than are those of the other workers. Hours of labor do not drag on the hands of those who are happy at their work.

This brings us to the next step in our description of the exact procedure that you must follow in developing initiative and leadership.

Second: You of course understand that the only way to get happiness is by giving it away, to others. The same applies to the development of initiative. You can best develop this essential quality in yourself by making it your business to interest those around you in doing the same. It is a well-known fact that a man learns best that which he endeavors to teach others. If a man embraces a certain creed or religious faith, the first thing he does is to go out and try to "sell" it to others. And in exact proportion to the extent to which he impresses others does he impress himself.

In the field of salesmanship it is a well-known fact that no salesman is successful in selling others until he has first made a good job of selling himself. Stated conversely, no salesman can do his best to sell others without sooner or later selling himself that which he is trying to sell to others.

Any statement that a person repeats over and over again for the purpose of inducing others to believe it, he, also, will come to believe, and this holds good whether the statement is false or true.

You can now see the advantage of making it your business to talk initiative, think initiative, eat initiative, sleep initiative and practice initiative. By so doing you are becoming a person of initiative and leadership, for it is a well-known fact that people will readily, willingly and voluntarily follow the person who shows by his actions that he is a person of initiative.

In the place where you work or the community in which you live you come in contact with other people. Make it your business to interest every one of them who will listen to you, in the development of initiative. It will not be necessary for you to give your reasons for doing this, nor will it be necessary for you to announce the fact that you are doing it. Just go ahead and do it. In your own mind you will understand, of course, that you are doing it because this practice will help you and will, at least, do those whom you influence in the same practice no harm.

If you wish to try an experiment that will prove both interesting and profitable to you, pick out some person of your acquaintance whom you know to be a person who never does anything that he is not expected to do, and begin selling him your idea of initiative. Do not stop by merely discussing the subject once; keep it up every time you have a convenient opportunity. Approach the subject from a different angle each time. If you go at this experiment in a tactful and forceful manner you will soon observe a change in the person on whom you are trying the experiment.

And, you will observe something else of more importance still: You will observe a change in yourself!

Do not fail to try this experiment.

You cannot talk initiative to others without developing a desire to practice it yourself. Through the operation of the principle of Auto-suggestion every statement that you make to others leaves its imprint on your own subconscious mind, and this holds good whether your statements are false or true.

You have often heard the saying: "He who lives by the sword will die by the sword."

Properly interpreted, this simply means that we are constantly attracting to ourselves and weaving into our own characters and personalities those qualities which our influence is helping to create in others. If we help others develop the habit of initiative, we, in turn, develop this same habit. If we sow the seeds of hatred and envy and discouragement in others, we, in turn, develop these qualities in ourselves. This principle through which a man comes to resemble in his own nature those whom he most admires is fully brought out in Hawthorne's story, The Great Stone Face, a story that every parent should have his offspring read.

We come, now, to the next step in our description of the exact procedure that you must follow in developing initiative and leadership.

Third: Before we go further let it be understood what is meant by the term "Leadership," as it is used in connection with this Reading Course on the Law of Success. There are two brands of leadership, and one of them is as deadly and destructive as the other is helpful and constructive. The deadly brand, which leads not to success, but to absolute failure, is the brand adopted by pseudo-leaders who force their leadership on unwilling followers. It will not be necessary here to describe this brand or to point out the fields of endeavor in which it is practiced, with the exception of the field of war, and in this field we will mention but one notable example, that of Napoleon.

Napoleon was a leader; there can be no doubt about this, but he led his followers and himself to destruction. The details are recorded in the history of France and the French people, where you may study them if you choose.

It is not Napoleon's brand of leadership that is recommended in this course, although I will admit that Napoleon possessed all the necessary fundamentals for great leadership, excepting one— he lacked the spirit of helpfulness to others as an objective. His desire for the power that comes through leadership was based solely upon self-aggrandizement. His desire for leadership was built upon personal ambition and not upon the desire to lift the French people to a higher and nobler station in the affairs of nations.

The brand of leadership that is recommended through this course of instruction is the brand which leads to self-determination and freedom and self-development and enlightenment and justice. This is the brand that endures. For example, and as a contrast with the brand of leadership through which Napoleon raised himself into prominence, consider our own American commoner, Lincoln. The object of his leadership was to bring truth and justice and understanding to the people of the United States. Even though he died a martyr to his belief in this brand of leadership, his name has been engraved upon the heart of the world in terms of loving kindliness that will never bring aught but good to the world.

Both Lincoln and Napoleon led armies in warfare, but the objects of their leadership were as different as night is different from day. If it would give you a better understanding of the principles upon which this Reading Course is based, you could easily be cited to leadership of today which resembles both the brand that Napoleon employed and that which Lincoln made the foundation of his life-work, but this is not essential; your own ability to look around and analyze men who take the leading parts in all lines of endeavor is sufficient to enable you to pick out the Lincoln as well as the Napoleon types. Your own judgment will help you decide which type you prefer to emulate.

There can be no doubt in your mind as to the brand of leadership that is recommended in this Reading Course, and there should be no question in your mind as to which of the two brands described you will adopt as your brand. We make no recommendations on this subject, however, for the reason that this Reading Course has been prepared as a means of laying before its students the fundamental principles upon which power is developed, and not as a preachment on ethical conduct. We present both the constructive and the destructive possibilities of the principles outlined in this course, that you may become familiar with both, but we leave entirely to your own discretion the choice and application of these principles, believing that your own intelligence will guide you to make a wise selection.

THE PENALTY OF LEADERSHIP

In every field of human endeavor, he that is first must perpetually live in the white light of publicity. Whether the leadership be vested in a man or in a manufactured product, emulation and envy are ever at work.

In art, in literature, in music, in industry, the reward and the punishment are always the same. The reward is widespread recognition; the punishments fierce denial and detraction.

When a man's work becomes a standard for the whole world, it also becomes a target for the shafts of the envious few. If his work be merely mediocre, he will be left severely alone—if he achieve a masterpiece, it will set a million tongues a-wagging.

Jealousy does not protrude its forked tongue at the artist who produces a commonplace painting.

Whatsoever you write, or paint, or play, or sing or build, no one will strive to surpass or slander you, unless your work be stamped with the seal of a genius.

Long, long after a great work or a good work has been done, those who are disappointed or envious continue to cry out that it cannot be done.

Mean voices were raised against the author of the Law of Success before the ink was dry on the first textbooks. Poisoned pens were released against both the author and the philosophy the moment the first edition of the course was printed.

Spiteful little voices in the domain of art were raised against our own Whistler as a mountebank, long after the big world acclaimed him its greatest artistic genius.

Multitudes flocked to Beyreuth to worship at the musical shrine of Wagner, while the little group of those whom he had dethroned and displaced argued angrily that he was no musician at all.

The little world continued to protest that Fulton could never build a steamboat, while the big world flocked to the river banks to see his boat steam by.

Small, narrow voices cried out that Henry Ford would not last another year, but above and beyond the din of their childish prattle Ford went silently about his business and made himself the richest and most powerful man on earth.

The leader is assailed because he is a leader, and the effort to equal him is merely added proof of his leadership.

Failing to equal or to excel, the follower seeks to depreciate and to destroy—but only confirms the superiority of that which he strives to supplant.

There is nothing new in this.

It is as old as the world and as old as the human passions—envy, fear, greed, ambition and the desire to surpass.

And it all avails nothing.

If the leader truly leads, he remains the LEADER!

Master-poet, master-painter, master-workman, each in his turn is assailed, and each holds his laurels through the ages.

That which is good or great makes itself known, no matter how loud the clamor of denial.

A real leader cannot be slandered or damaged by lies of the envious, because all such attempts serve only to turn the spotlight on his ability, and real ability always finds a generous following.

Attempts to destroy real Leadership is love's labor lost, because that which deserves to live, lives!

◆

We come back, now, to the discussion of the third step of the procedure that you must follow in developing initiative and leadership. This third step takes us back for a review of the principle of organized effort, as described in the preceding lessons of this course.

You have already learned that no man can accomplish enduring results of a far-reaching nature without the aid and cooperation of others. You have already learned that when two or more persons ally themselves in any undertaking, in a spirit of harmony and understanding, each person in the alliance thereby multiplies his own powers of achievement. Nowhere is this principle more evidenced than it is in an industry or business in which there is perfect teamwork between the employer and the employees. Wherever you find this teamwork you find prosperity and goodwill on both sides.

Co-operation is said to be the most important word in the English language. It plays an important part in the affairs of the home, in the relationship of man and wife, parents and children. It plays an important part in the affairs of state. So important is this principle of co-operation that no leader can become powerful or last long who does not understand and apply it in his leadership.

Lack of Co-operation has destroyed more business enterprises than have all other causes combined. In my twenty-five years of active business experience and observation I have witnessed the destruction of all manner of business enterprises because of dissension and lack of application of this principle of Cooperation. In the practice of law I have observed the destruction of homes and divorce cases without end as a result of the lack of Co-operation between man and wife. In the study of the histories of nations it becomes alarmingly obvious that lack of Co-operative effort has been a curse to the human race all back down the ages. Turn back the pages of these histories and study them and you will learn a lesson in Co-operation, that will impress itself indelibly upon your mind.

You are paying, and your children and your children's children will continue to pay, for the cost of the most expensive and destructive war the world has ever known, because nations have not yet learned that a part of the world cannot suffer without damage and suffering to the whole world.

This same rule applies, with telling effect, in the conduct of modern business and industry. When an industry becomes disorganized and torn asunder by strikes and other forms of disagreement, both the employers and employees suffer irreparable loss. But, the damage does not stop here; this loss becomes a burden to the public and takes on the form of higher prices and scarcity of the necessities of life.

The people of the United States who rent their homes are feeling the burden, at this very moment, of lack of co-operation between contractors and builders and the workers. So uncertain has the relationship between the contractors and their employees become that the contractors will not undertake a building without adding to the cost an arbitrary sum sufficient to protect them in the event of labor troubles. This additional cost increases rents and places unnecessary burdens upon the backs of millions of people. In this instance the lack of co-operation between a few men places heavy and almost unbearable burdens upon millions of people.

The same evil exists in the operation of our railroads. Lack of harmony and co-operation between the railroad management and the workers has made it necessary for the railroads to increase their freight and passenger rates, and this, in turn, has increased the cost of life's necessities to almost unbearable proportions. Here, again, lack of co-operation between a few leads to hardship for millions of people.

These facts are cited without effort or desire to place the responsibility for this lack of co-operation, since the object of this Reading Course is to help its students get at facts.

It may be truthfully stated that the high cost of living that everywhere manifests itself today has grown out of lack of application of the principle of co-operative leadership. Those who wish to decry present systems of government and industrial management may do so, but in the final analysis it becomes obvious to all except those who are not seeking the truth that the evils of government and of industry have grown out of lack of co-operation.

Nor can it be truthfully said that all the evils of the world are confined to the affairs of state and industry. Take a look at the churches and you will observe the damaging effects of lack of cooperation. No particular church is cited, but analyze any church or group of churches where lack of co-ordination of effort prevails and you will see evidence of disintegration that limits the service those churches could render. For example, take the average town or small city where rivalry has sprung up between the churches and notice what has happened; especially those towns in which the number of churches is far out of proportion to the population.

Through harmonized effort and through cooperation, the churches of the world could wield sufficient influence to render war an impossibility. Through this same principle of co-operative effort the churches and the leaders of business and industry could eliminate rascality and sharp practices, and all this could be brought about speedily.

These possibilities are not mentioned in a spirit of criticism, but only as a means of illustrating the power of co-operation, and to emphasize my belief in the potential power of the churches of the world. So there will be no possibility of misinterpretation of my meaning in the reference that I have here made to the churches I will repeat that which I have so often said in person;

namely, that had it not been for the influence of the churches no man would be safe in walking down the street. Men would be at each other's throat like wolves and civilization would still be in the pre-historic age. My complaint is not against the work that the churches have done, but the work that they could have done through leadership that was based upon the principle of co-ordinated, co-operative effort which would have carried civilization at least a thousand years ahead of where it is today. It is not yet too late for such leadership.

That you may more fully grasp the fundamental principle of co-operative effort you are urged to go to the public library and read *The Science of Power*, by Benjamin Kidd. Out of scores of volumes by some of the soundest thinkers of the world that I have read during the past fifteen years, no single volume has given me such a full understanding of the possibilities of co-operative effort as has this book. In recommending that you read this book it is not my purpose to endorse the book in its entirety, for it offers some theories with which I am not in accord. If you read it, do so with an open mind and take from it only that which you feel you can use to advantage in achieving the object of your definite chief aim. The book will stimulate thought, which is the greatest service that any book can render. As a matter of fact the chief object of this Reading Course on the Law of Success is to stimulate deliberate thought: particularly that brand of thought that is free from bias and prejudice and is seeking truth no matter where or how or when it may be found.

During the World War I was fortunate enough to listen to a great soldier's analysis of how to be a leader. This analysis was given to the student-officers of the Second Training Camp at Fort Sheridan, by Major C. A. Bach, a quiet, unassuming army officer acting as an instructor. I have preserved a copy of this address because I believe it to be one of the finest lessons on leadership ever recorded.

The wisdom of Major Bach's address is so vital to the business man aspiring to leadership, or to the section boss, or to the stenographer, or to the foreman of the shop, or to the president of the works, that I have preserved it as a part of this Reading Course. It is my earnest hope that through the agency of this course this remarkable dissertation on leadership will find its way into the hands of every employer and every worker and every ambitious person who aspires to leadership in any walk of life. The principles upon which the address is based are as applicable to leadership in business and industry and finance as they are in the successful conduct of warfare.

Major Bach spoke as follows:

In a short time each of you men will control the lives of a certain number of other men. You will have in your charge loyal but untrained citizens, who look to you for instruction and guidance. Your word will be their law. Your most casual remark will be remembered. Your mannerisms will be aped. Your clothing, your carriage, your vocabulary, your manner of command will be imitated.

When you join your organization you will find there a willing body of men who ask from you nothing more than the qualities that will command their respect, their loyalty and their obedience.

They are perfectly ready and eager to follow you so long as you can convince them that you have these qualities. When the time comes that they are satisfied you do not possess them you might as well kiss yourself goodbye. Your usefulness in that organization is at an end.

[How remarkably true this is in all manner of leadership.]

From the standpoint of society, the world may be divided

into leaders and followers. The professions have their leaders, the financial world has its leaders. In all this leadership it is difficult, if not impossible, to separate from the element of pure leadership that selfish element of personal gain or advantage to the individual, without which any leadership would lose its value.

It is in military service only, where men freely sacrifice their lives for a faith, where men are willing to suffer and die for the right or the prevention of a wrong, that we can hope to realize leadership in its most exalted and disinterested sense. Therefore, when I say leadership, I mean military leadership.

In a few days the great mass of you men will receive commissions as officers. These commissions will not make you leaders; they will merely make you officers. They will place you in a position where you can become leaders if you possess the proper attributes. But you must make good, not so much with the men over you as with the men under you.

Men must and will follow into battle officers who are not leaders, but the driving power behind these men is not enthusiasm but discipline. They go with doubt and trembling that prompts the unspoken question, "What will he do next?" Such men obey the letter of their orders but no more. Of devotion to their commander, of exalted enthusiasm which scorns personal risk, of self-sacrifice to insure his personal safety, they know nothing. Their legs carry them forward because their brain and their training tell them they must go. Their spirit does not go with them.

Great results are not achieved by cold, passive, unresponsive soldiers. They don't go very far and they stop as soon as they can. leadership not only demands but receives the willing, unhesitating, unfaltering obedience and loyalty of other men; and a devotion that will cause them, when the time comes, to follow their uncrowned king to hell and back again, if necessary.

You will ask yourselves: "Of just what, then, does leadership consist? What must I do to become a leader? What are the attributes of leadership, and how can I cultivate them?"

Leadership is a composite of a number of qualities. [Just as success is a composite of the fifteen factors out of which this Reading Course was built.] Among the most important I would list Self-confidence, Moral Ascendency, Self-Sacrifice, Paternalism, Fairness, Initiative, Decision, Dignity, Courage.

Self-confidence results, first, from exact knowledge; second, the ability to impart that knowledge; and third, the feeling of superiority over others that naturally follows. All these give the officer poise. To lead, you must know! You may bluff all of your men some of the time, but you can't do it all the time. Men will not have confidence in an officer unless he knows his business, and he must know it from the ground up.

The officer should know more about paper work than his first sergeant and company clerk put together; he should know more about messing than his mess sergeant; more about diseases of the horse than his troop farrier. He should be at least as good a shot as any man in his company.

If the officer does not know, and demonstrates the fact that he does not know, it is entirely human for the soldier to say to himself, "To hell with him. He doesn't know as much about this as I do," and calmly disregard the instructions received.

There is no substitute for accurate knowledge!

Become so well informed that men will hunt you up to ask questions; that your brother officers will say to one another, "Ask Smith—he knows."

And not only should each officer know thoroughly the duties of his own grade, but he should study those of the two grades next above him. A twofold benefit attaches to this.

He prepares himself for duties which may fall to his lot any time during battle; he further gains a broader viewpoint which enables him to appreciate the necessity for the issuance of orders and join more intelligently in their execution.

Not only must the officer know but he must be able to put what he knows into grammatical, interesting, forceful English. He must learn to stand on his feet and speak without embarrassment.

I am told that in British training camps student-officers are required to deliver ten minute talks on any subject they choose. That is excellent practice. For to speak clearly one must think clearly, and clear, logical thinking expresses itself in definite, positive orders.

While self-confidence is the result of knowing more than your men, Moral Ascendency over them is based upon your belief that you are the better man. To gain and maintain this ascendency you must have self-control, physical vitality and endurance and moral force. You must have yourself so well in hand that, even though in battle you be scared stiff, you will never show fear. For if by so much as a hurried movement or a trembling of the hands, or a change of expression, or a hasty order hastily revoked, you indicate your mental condition it will be reflected in your men in a far greater degree.

In garrison or camp many instances will arise to try your temper and wreck the sweetness of your disposition. If at such times you "fly off the handle" you have no business to be in charge of men. For men in anger say and do things that they almost invariably regret afterward.

An officer should never apologize to bis men; also an officer should never he guilty of an act for which his sense of justice tells him he should apologize.

Another element in gaining Moral Ascendency lies in

the possession of enough physical vitality and endurance to withstand the hardships to which you and your men are subjected, and a dauntless spirit that enables you not only to accept them cheerfully but to minimize their magnitude.

Make light of your troubles, belittle your trials and you will help vitally to build up within your organization an esprit whose value in time of stress cannot be measured.

Moral force is the third element in gaining Moral Ascendency. To exert moral force you must live clean; you must have sufficient brain power to see the right and the will to do right.

Be an example to your men!

An officer can be a power for good or a power for evil. Don't preach to them—that will be worse than useless. Live the kind of life you would have them lead, and you will be surprised to see the number that will imitate you.

A loud-mouthed, profane captain who is careless of his personal appearance will have a loud-mouthed, profane, dirty company. Remember what I tell you. Your company will he the reflection of yourself. If you have a rotten company it will be because you are a rotten captain.

Self-sacrifice is essential to leadership. You will give, give, all the time. You will give of yourself physically, for the longest hours, the hardest work and the greatest responsibility are the lot of the captain. He is the first man up in the morning and the last man in at night. He works while others sleep.

You will give of yourself mentally, in sympathy and appreciation for the troubles of men in your charge. This one's mother has died, and that one has lost all his savings in a bank failure. They may desire help, but more than anything else they desire sympathy. Don't make the mistake of turning such men down with the statement that you have troubles of your own, for every time you do that you knock a stone out of the foundation of your house.

Your men are your foundation, and your house of leadership will tumble about your ears unless it rests securely upon them. Finally, you will give of your own slender financial resources. You will frequently spend your own money to conserve the health and well-being of your men or to assist them when in trouble. Generally you get your money back. Very frequently you must charge it off to profit and loss.

Even so, it is worth the cost.

When I say that paternalism is essential to leadership I use the term in its better sense. I do not now refer to that form of paternalism which robs men of initiative, self-reliance and self-respect. I refer to the paternalism that manifests itself in a watchful care for the comfort and welfare of those in your charge.

Soldiers are much like children. You must see that they have shelter, food and clothing, the best that your utmost efforts can provide. You must see that they have food to eat before you think of your own; that they have each as good a bed as can be provided before you consider where you will sleep. You must be far more solicitous of their comfort than of your own. You must look after their health. You must conserve their strength by not demanding needless exertion or useless labor.

And by doing all these things you are breathing life into what would be otherwise a mere machine. You are creating a soul in your organization that will make the mass respond to you as though it were one man. And that is esprit.

And when your organization has this esprit you will wake up some morning and discover that the tables have been turned; that instead of your constantly looking out for them they have, without even a hint from you, taken up the task of looking out for you. You will find that a detail is always there to see that your tent, if you have one, is promptly pitched; that the most and the cleanest bedding is brought to your tent; that from some mysterious source two eggs have been added to your supper when no one else has any; that an extra man is helping your men give your horse a super grooming; that your wishes are anticipated; that every man is "Johnny-on-the-spot." And then you have arrived!

You cannot treat all men alike! A punishment that would be dismissed by one man with a shrug of the shoulders is mental anguish for another. A company commander who, for a given offense, has a standard punishment that applies to all is either too indolent or too stupid to study the personality of his men. In his case justice is certainly blind.

Study your men as carefully as a surgeon studies a difficult case. And when you are sure of your diagnosis apply the remedy. And remember that you apply the remedy to effect a cure, not merely to see the victim squirm. It may be necessary to cut deep, but when you are satisfied as to your diagnosis don't be diverted from your purpose by any false sympathy for the patient.

Hand in hand with fairness in awarding punishment walks fairness in giving credit. Everybody hates a human hog. When one of your men has accomplished an especially creditable piece of work see that he gets the proper reward. Turn heaven and earth upside down to get it for him. Don't try to take it away from him and hog it for yourself. You may do this and get away with it, but you have lost the respect and loyalty of your men. Sooner or later your brother officers will hear of it and shun you like a leper. In war there is glory enough for all. Give the man under you his due. The man who always takes and never gives is not a leader. He is a parasite.

There is another kind of fairness—that which will prevent an officer from abusing the privileges of his rank. When you exact respect from soldiers be sure you treat them with equal respect. Build up their manhood and self-respect. Don't try to pull it down.

For an officer to be overbearing and insulting in the treatment of enlisted men is the act of a coward. He ties the man to a tree with the ropes of discipline and then strikes him in the face knowing full well that the man cannot strike back.

Consideration, courtesy and respect from officers toward enlisted men are not incompatible with discipline. They are parts of our discipline. Without initiative and decision no man can expect to lead.

In maneuvers you will frequently see, when an emergency arises, certain men calmly give instant orders which later, on analysis, prove to be, if not exactly the right thing, very nearly the right thing to have done. You will see other men in emergency become badly rattled; their brains refuse to work, or they give a hasty order, revoke it; give another, revoke that; in short, show every indication of being in a blue funk.

Regarding the first man you may say: "That man is a genius. He hasn't had time to reason this thing out. He acts intuitively." Forget it! Genius is merely the capacity for taking infinite pains. The man who was ready is the man who has prepared himself. He has studied beforehand the possible situations that might arise; he has made tentative plans covering such situations. When he is confronted by the emergency he is ready to meet it. He must have sufficient mental alertness to appreciate the problem that confronts him and the power of quick reasoning to determine what changes are necessary in his already formulated plan. He must also have the decision to order the execution and stick to his orders.

Any reasonable order in an emergency is better than no order. The situation is there. Meet it. It is better to do something and do the wrong thing than to hesitate, hunt around for the right thing to do and wind up by doing nothing at all. And, having decided on a line of action, stick to it. Don't vacillate. Men have no confidence in an officer who doesn't know his own mind.

Occasionally you will be called upon to meet a situation which no reasonable human being could anticipate. If you have prepared yourself to meet other emergencies which you could anticipate, the mental training you have thereby gained will enable you to act promptly and with calmness.

You must frequently act without orders from higher authority. Time will not permit you to wait for them. Here again enters the importance of studying the work of officers above you. If you have a comprehensive grasp of the entire situation and can form an idea of the general plan of your superiors, that and your previous emergency training will enable you to determine that the responsibility is yours and to issue the necessary orders without delay.

The element of personal dignity is important in military leadership. Be the friend of your men, but do not become their intimate. Your men should stand in awe of you—not fear! If your men presume to become familiar it is your fault, and not theirs. Your actions have encouraged them to do so. And, above all things, don't cheapen yourself by courting their friendship or currying their favor. They will despise: you for it. If you are worthy of their loyalty and respect and devotion they will surely give all these without asking. If you are not, nothing that you can do will win them.

It is exceedingly difficult for an officer to be dignified while wearing a dirty, spotted uniform and a three days' stubble of whiskers on his face. Such a man lacks self-respect, and self-respect is an essential of dignity.

There may be occasions when your work entails dirty clothes and an unshaved face. Your men all look that way. At such times there is ample reason for your appearance. In fact, it would be a mistake to look too clean—they would think that you were, not doing your share. But as soon as this unusual occasion has passed set an example for personal neatness.

And then I would mention courage. Moral courage you need as well as mental courage—that kind of moral courage which enables you to adhere without faltering to a determined course of action, which your judgment has indicated is the one best suited to secure the desired results.

You will find many times, especially in action, that, after having issued your orders to do a certain thing, you will be beset by misgivings and doubts; you will see, or think you see, other and better means for accomplishing the object sought. You will be strongly tempted to change your orders. Don't do it until it is clearly manifested that your first orders were radically wrong. For, if you do, you will be again worried by doubts as to the efficacy of your second orders.

Every time you change your orders without obvious reason you weaken your authority and impair the confidence of your men. Have the moral courage to stand by your order and see it through.

Moral courage further demands that you assume the responsibility for your own acts. If your subordinates have loyally carried out your orders and the movement you directed is a failure the failure is yours, not theirs. Yours would have been the honor had it been successful. Take the blame if it results in disaster. Don't try to shift it to a subordinate and make him the goat. That is a cowardly act. Furthermore, you will need moral courage to determine the fate of those under you. You will frequently be called upon for recommendations for promotion or demotion of officers and noncommissioned officers in your immediate command.

Keep clearly in mind your personal integrity and the duty you owe your country. Do not let yourself be deflected from a strict sense of justice by feelings of personal friendship. If your own brother is your second lieutenant, and you find him unfit to hold his commission, eliminate him. If you don't your lack of moral courage may result in the loss of valuable lives.

If, on the other hand, you are called upon for a recommendation concerning a man whom, for personal reasons, you thoroughly dislike, do not fail to do him full justice. Remember that your aim is the general good, not the satisfaction of an individual grudge.

I am taking it for granted that you have physical courage. I need not tell you how necessary that is. Courage is more than bravery. Bravery is fearlessness—the absence of fear. The merest dolt may be brave, because he lacks the mentality to appreciate his danger; he doesn't know enough to be afraid.

Courage, however, is that firmness of spirit, that moral backbone which, while fully appreciating the danger involved, nevertheless goes on with the undertaking. Bravery is physical; courage is mental and moral. You may be cold all over; your hands may tremble; your legs may quake; your knees be ready to give way—that is fear. If, nevertheless, you go forward; if, in spite of this physical defection you continue to lead your men against the enemy, you have courage. The physical manifestations of fear will pass away. You may never experience them but once. They are the "buck fever" of the hunter who tries to shoot his first deer. You must not give way to them.

A number of years ago, while taking a course in demolitions, the class of which I was a member was handling dynamite. The instructor said, regarding its manipulation: "I must caution you gentlemen to be careful in the use of these explosives. One man has but one accident." And so I would caution you. If you give way to fear that will doubtless beset you in your first action; if you show the white feather; if you let your men go forward while you hunt a shell crater, you will never again have the opportunity of leading those men.

Use judgment in calling on your men for displays of physical courage or bravery. Don't ask any man to go where you would not go yourself. If your common sense tells you that the place is too dangerous for you to venture into, then it is too dangerous for him. You know his life is as valuable to him as yours is to you.

Occasionally some of your men must be exposed to danger which you cannot share. A message must be taken across a fire-swept zone. You call for volunteers. If your men know you and know that you are "right" you will never lack volunteers, for they will know your heart is in your work, that you are giving your country the best you have, that you would willingly carry the message yourself if you could. Your example and enthusiasm will have inspired them.

And, lastly, if you aspire to leadership, I would urge you to study men.

Get under their skins and find out what is inside. Some men are quite different from what they appear to be on the surface. Determine the workings of their mind.

Much of General Robert E. Tee's success as a leader may be ascribed to his ability as a psychologist. He knew most of his opponents from West Point days; knew the workings of their minds; and he believed that they would do certain things under certain circumstances. In nearly every case he was able to anticipate their movements and block the execution.

You cannot know your opponent in this war in the same

way. But you can know your own men. You can study each to determine wherein lies his strength and his weakness; which man can be relied upon to the last gasp and which cannot.

Know your men, know your business, know yourself!

◆

In all literature you will not find a better description of leadership than this. Apply it to yourself, or to your business, or to your profession, or to the place where you are employed, and you will observe how well it serves as your guide.

Major Bach's address is one that might well be delivered to every boy and girl who graduates in high school. It might well be delivered to every college graduate. It might well become the book of rules for every man who is placed in a position of leadership over other men, no matter in what calling, business or profession.

In Lesson Two you learned the value of a definite chief aim. Let it be here emphasized that your aim must be active and not passive. A definite aim will never be anything else but a mere wish unless you become a person of initiative and aggressively and persistently pursue that aim until it has been fulfilled.

You can get nowhere without persistence, a fact which cannot be too often repeated.

The difference between persistence and lack of it is the same as the difference between wishing for a thing and positively determining to get it.

To become a person of initiative you must form the habit of aggressively and persistently following the object of your definite chief aim until you acquire it, whether this requires one year or twenty years. You might as well have no definite chief aim as to have such an aim without continuous effort to achieve it.

You are not making the most of this course if you do not

take some step each day that brings you nearer realization of your definite chief aim. Do not fool yourself, or permit yourself to be misled to believe that the object of your definite chief aim will matter—alive if you only wait. The materialization will come through your own determination, backed by your own carefully laid plans and your own initiative in putting those plans into action, or it will not come at all.

One of the major requisites for Leadership is the power of quick and firm DECISION!

Analysis of more than 16,000 people disclosed the fact that Leaders are always men of ready decision, even in matters of small importance, while the follower is NEVER a person of quick decision.

This is worth remembering!

The follower, in whatever walk of life you find him, is a man who seldom knows what he wants. He vacillates, procrastinates, and actually refuses to reach a decision, even in matters of the smallest importance, unless a Leader induces him to do so.

To know that the majority of people cannot and will not reach decisions quickly, if at all, is of great help to the Leader who knows what he wants and has a plan for getting it.

Here it will be observed how closely allied are the two laws covered by Lesson Two and this lesson. The Leader not only works with A DEFINITE CHIEF AIM, but he has a very definite plan for attaining the object of that aim. It will be seen, also, that the Law of Self-confidence becomes an important part of the working equipment of the Leader.

The chief reason why the follower does not reach decisions is that he lacks the Self-confidence to do so. Every Leader makes use of the Law of a Definite Purpose, the Law of Self-confidence and the Law of Initiative and Leadership. And if he is an outstanding, successful Leader he makes use, also, of the Laws of Imagination, Enthusiasm, Self-Control, Pleasing Personality, Accurate Thinking, Concentration and Tolerance. Without the combined use of all these Laws no one may become a really great Leader. Omission of a single one of these Laws lessens the power of the Leader proportionately.

A salesman for the LaSalle Extension University called on a real estate dealer, in a small western town, for the purpose of trying to sell the real estate man a course in Salesmanship and Business Management.

When the salesman arrived at the prospective student's office he found the gentleman pecking out a letter by the two-finger method, on an antiquated typewriter. The salesman introduced himself, then proceeded to state his business and describe the course he had come to sell.

The real estate man listened with apparent interest.

After the sales talk had been completed the salesman hesitated, waiting for some signs of "yes" or "no" from his prospective client. Thinking that perhaps he had not made the sales talk quite strong enough, he briefly went over the merits of the course he was selling, a second time. Still there was no response from the prospective student.

The salesman then asked the direct question, "You want this course, do you not?"

In a slow, drawling tone of voice, the real estate man replied:

"Well, I hardly know whether I do or not."

No doubt he was telling the truth, because he was one of the millions of men who find it hard to reach decisions.

Being an able judge of human nature the salesman then arose, put on his hat, placed his literature back in his brief case and made ready to leave. Then he resorted to tactics which were somewhat drastic, and took the real estate man by surprise with this startling statement:

"I am going to take it upon myself to say something to you that you will not like, but it may be of help to you.

"Take a look at this office in which you work! The floor is dirty; the walls are dusty; the typewriter you are using looks as if it might be the one Mr. Noah used in the Ark during the big flood; your pants are bagged at the knees; your collar is dirty; your face is unshaved, and you have a look in your eyes that tells me you are defeated.

"Please go ahead and get mad—that's just what I want you to do, because it may shock you into doing some thinking that will be helpful to you and to those who are dependent upon you.

"I can see, in my imagination, the home in which you live. Several little children, none too well dressed, and perhaps none too well fed; a mother whose dress is three seasons out of style, whose eyes carry the same look of defeat that yours do. This little woman whom you married has stuck by you but you have not made good in life as she had hoped, when you were first married, that you would.

"Please remember that I am not now talking to a prospective student, because I would not sell you this course at THIS PARTICULAR MOMENT if you offered to pay cash in advance, because if I did you would not have the initiative to complete it, and we want no failures on our student list.

"The talk I am now giving you will make it impossible, perhaps, for me ever to sell you anything, but it is going to do something for you that has never been done before, providing it makes you think.

"Now, I will tell you in a very few words exactly why you are defeated; why you are pecking out letters on an old typewriter, in an old dirty office, in a little town: IT IS BECAUSE YOU DO NOT HAVE THE POWER TO REACH A DECISION!

"All your life you have been forming the habit of dodging the responsibility of reaching decisions, until you have come, now, to where it is well-nigh impossible for you to do so.

"If you had told me that you wanted the course, or that you did not want it, I could have sympathized with you, because I would have known that lack of funds was what caused you to hesitate, but what did you say? Why, you admitted you did not know whether you wanted it or not.

"If you will think over what I have said I am sure you will acknowledge that it has become a habit with you to dodge the responsibility of reaching clear-cut decisions on practically all matters that affect you."

The real estate man sat glued in his chair, with his under jaw dropped, his eyes bulged in astonishment, but he made no attempt to answer the biting indictment.

The salesman said goodbye and started for the door.

After he had closed the door behind him he again opened it, walked back in, with a smile on his face, took his seat in front of the astonished real estate man, and explained his conduct in this way:

"I do not blame you at all if you feel hurt at my remarks. In fact I sort of hope that you have been offended, but now let me say this, man to man, that I think you have intelligence and I am sure you have ability, but you have fallen into a habit that has whipped you. No man is ever down and out until he is under the sod. You may be temporarily down, but you can get up again, and I am just sportsman enough to give you my hand and offer you a lift, if you will accept my apologies for what I have said.

"You do not belong in this town. You would starve to death in the real estate business in this place, even if you were a Leader in your field. Get yourself a new suit of clothes, even if you have to borrow the money with which to do it, then go over to St. Louis with me and I will introduce you to a real estate man who will give you a chance to earn some money and at the same time teach you some of the important things about this line of work that you can capitalize later on.

"If you haven't enough credit to get the clothes you need I will stand good for you at a store in St. Louis where I have a charge account. I am in earnest and my offer to help you is based upon the highest motive that can actuate a human being. I am successful in my own field, but I have not always been so. I went through just what you are now going through, but, the important thing is that I WENT THROUGH IT, and got it over with, JUST AS YOU ARE GOING TO DO IF YOU WILL FOLLOW MY ADVICE.

"Will you come with me?"

The real estate man started to arise, but his legs wobbled and he sank back into his chair. Despite the fact that he was a great big fellow, with rather pronounced manly qualities, known as the "he-man" type, his emotions got the better of him and he actually wept.

He made a second attempt and got on his feet, shook hands with the salesman, thanked him for his kindness, and said he was going to follow the advice, but he would do so in his own way.

Calling for an application blank he signed for the course on Salesmanship and Business Management, made the first payment in nickels and dimes, and told the salesman he would hear from him again.

Three years later this real estate man had an organization of sixty salesmen, and one of the most successful real estate businesses in the city of St. Louis. The author of this course (who was advertising manager of the LaSalle Extension University at the time this incident happened) has been in this real estate man's office many times and has observed him over a period of more than fifteen years. He is an entirely different man from the person interviewed by the LaSalle salesman over fifteen years ago, and the thing that made him different is the same that will make YOU different: it is the power of DECISION which is so essential to Leadership.

This real estate man is now a Leader in the real estate field. He is directing the efforts of other salesmen and helping them to become more efficient. This one change in his philosophy has turned temporary defeat into success. Every new salesman who goes to work for this man is called into his private office, before he is employed, and told the story of his own transformation, word for word just as it occurred when the LaSalle salesman first met him in his shabby little real estate office.

◆

Some eighteen years ago the author of this course made his first trip to the little town of Lumberport, W. Va. At that time the only means of transportation leading from Clarksburg, the largest nearby center, to Lumberport, was the Baltimore & Ohio Railroad and an interurban electric line which ran within three miles of the town; one could walk the three miles if he chose.

Upon arrival at Clarksburg I found that the only train going to Lumberport in the forenoon had already gone, and not wishing to wait for the later afternoon train I made the trip by trolley, with the intention of walking the three miles. On the way down the rain began to pour, and those three miles had to be navigated on foot, through deep yellow mud. When I arrived at Lumberport my shoes and pants were muddy, and my disposition was none the better for the experience.

The first person I met was V. L. Hornor, who was then

cashier of the Lumberport Bank. In a rather loud tone of voice I asked of him, "Why do you not get that trolley line extended from the junction over to Lumberport so your friends can get in and out of town without drowning in mud?"

"Did you see a river with high banks, at the edge of the town, as you came in?" he asked. I replied that I had seen it. "Well," he continued, "that's the reason we have no street cars running into town. The cost of a bridge would be about $100,000.00, and that is more than the company owning the trolley line is willing to invest. We have been trying for ten years to get them to build a line into town."

"Trying!" I exploded. "How hard have you tried?"

"We have offered them every inducement we could afford, such as free right of way from the junction into the town, and free use of the streets, but that bridge is the stumbling block. They simply will not stand the expense. Claim they cannot afford such an expense for the small amount of revenue they would receive from the three mile extension."

Then the Law of Success philosophy began to come to my rescue!

I asked Mr. Hornor if he would take a walk over to the river with me, that we might look at the spot that was causing so much inconvenience. He said he would be glad to do so.

When we got to the river I began to take inventory of everything in sight. I observed that the Baltimore & Ohio Railroad tracks ran up and down the river banks, on both sides of the river; that the county road crossed the river on a rickety wooden bridge, both approaches to which were over several strands of railroad track, as the railroad company had its switching yards at that point.

While we were standing there a freight train blocked the crossing and several teams stopped on both sides of the train, waiting for an opportunity to get through. The train kept the road blocked for about twenty-five minutes.

With this combination of circumstances in mind it required but little imagination to see that THREE DIFFERENT PARTIES were or could be interested in the building of the bridge such as would be needed to carry the weight of a street car.

It was obvious that the Baltimore & Ohio Railroad Company would be interested in such a bridge, because that would remove the county road from their switching tracks, and save them a possible accident on the crossing, to say nothing of much loss of time and expense in cutting trains to allow teams to pass.

It was also obvious that the County Commissioners would be interested in the bridge, because it would raise the county road to a better level and make it more serviceable to the public. And, of course the street railway company was interested in the bridge, but IT DID NOT WISH TO PAY THE ENTIRE COST.

All these facts passed through my mind as I stood there and watched the freight train being cut for the traffic to pass through.

A DEFINITE CHIEF AIM took place in my mind. Also, a definite plan for its attainment. The next day I got together a committee of townspeople, consisting of the mayor, councilmen and some leading citizens, and called on the Division Superintendent of the Baltimore & Ohio Railroad Company, at Grafton. We convinced him that it was worth one third of the cost of the bridge to get the county road off his company's tracks. Next we went to the County Commissioners and found them to be quite enthusiastic over the possibility of getting a new bridge by paying for only one third of it. They promised to pay their one third providing we could arrange for the other two thirds.

We then went to the president of the Traction Company that owned the trolley line, at Fairmont, and laid before him an offer to donate all the rights of way and pay for two thirds of the cost of the bridge providing he would begin building the line into town promptly. We found him receptive, also.

Three weeks later a contract had been signed between the Baltimore & Ohio Railroad Company, the Monongahela Valley Traction Company and the County Commissioners of Harrison County, providing for the construction of the bridge, one third of its cost to be paid by each.

Two months later the right of way was being graded and the bridge was under way, and three months after that street cars were running into Lumberport on regular schedule.

This incident meant much to the town of Lumberport, because it provided transportation that enabled people to get in and out of the town without undue effort.

It also meant a great deal to me, because it served to introduce me as one who "got things done." Two very definite advantages resulted from this transaction. The Chief Counsel for the Traction Company gave me a position as his assistant, and later on it was the means of an introduction which led to my appointment as the advertising manager of the LaSalle Extension University.

Lumberport, W. Va., was then, and still is a small town, and Chicago was a large city and located a considerable distance away, but news of Initiative and Leadership has a way of taking on wings and traveling.

Four of the Fifteen Laws of Success were combined in the transaction described, namely: A DEFINITE CHIEF AIM, SELF-CONFIDENCE, IMAGINATION and INITIATIVE and LEADERSHIP. The Law of DOING MORE THAN PAID

FOR also entered, somewhat, into the transaction, because I was not offered anything and in fact did not expect pay for what I did.

To be perfectly frank I appointed myself to the job of getting the bridge built more as a sort of challenge to those who said it could not be done than I did with the expectation of getting paid for it. By my attitude I rather intimated to Mr. Hornor that I could get the job done, and he was not slow to snap me up and put me to the test.

It may be helpful to call attention here to the part which IMAGINATION played in this transaction. For ten years the townspeople of Lumberport had been trying to get a street car line built into town. It must not be concluded that the town was without men of ability, because that would be inaccurate. In fact there were many men of ability in the town, but they had been making the mistake which is so commonly made by us all, of trying to solve their problem through one single source, whereas there were actually THREE SOURCES of solution available to them.

$100,000.00 was too much for one company to assume, for the construction of a bridge, but when the cost was distributed between three interested parties the amount to be borne by each was more reasonable.

The question might be asked: "Why did not some of the local townsmen think of this three-way solution?"

In the first place they were so close to their problem that they failed to take a perspective, bird's-eye view of it, which would have suggested the solution. This, also, is a common mistake, and one that is always avoided by great Leaders. In the second place these townspeople had never before co-ordinated their efforts or worked as an organized group with the sole purpose in mind of finding a way to get a street car line built into town. This, also, is another common error made by men in all walks of life—that of failure to work in unison, in a thorough spirit of co-operation.

I, being an outsider, had less difficulty in getting co-operative action than one of their own group might have had. Too often there is a spirit of selfishness in small communities which prompts each individual to think that his ideas should prevail. It is an important part of the Leader's responsibility to induce people to subordinate their own ideas and interests for the good of the whole, and this applies to matters of a civic, business, social, political, financial or industrial nature.

Success, no matter what may be one's conception of that term, is nearly always a question of one's ability to get others to subordinate their own individualities and follow a Leader. The Leader who has the Personality and the Imagination to induce his followers to accept his plans and carry them out faithfully is always an able Leader.

The next lesson, on IMAGINATION, will take you still further into the art of tactful Leadership. In fact Leadership and Imagination are so closely allied and so essential for success that one cannot be successfully applied without the other. Initiative is the moving force that pushes the Leader ahead, but Imagination is the guiding spirit that tells him which way to go.

Imagination enabled the author of this course to analyze the Lumberport bridge problem, break it up into its three component parts, and assemble these parts in a practical working plan. Nearly every problem may be so broken up into parts which are more easily managed, as parts, than they are when assembled as a whole. Perhaps one of the most important advantages of Imagination is that it enables one to separate all problems into their component parts and to reassemble them in more favorable combinations.

It has been said that all battles in warfare are won or lost, not on the firing line, after the battle begins, but back of the lines, through the sound strategy, or the lack of it, used by the generals who plan the battles.

What is true of warfare is equally true in business, and in most other problems which confront us throughout life. We win or lose according to the nature of the plans we build and carry out, a fact which serves to emphasize the value of the Laws of Initiative and Leadership, Imagination, Self-confidence and a Definite Chief Aim. With the intelligent use of these four laws one may build plans, for any purpose whatsoever, which cannot be defeated by any person or group of persons who do not employ or understand these laws.

There is no escape from the truth here stated!

ORGANIZED EFFORT is effort which is directed according to a plan that was conceived with the aid of Imagination, guided by a Definite Chief Aim, and given momentum with Initiative and Self-confidence. These four laws blend into one and become a power in the hands of a Leader. Without their aid effective leadership is impossible.

6

—

SETTING GOALS

Dale Carnegie

At age twenty-three I was one of the unhappiest young men in New York. I was selling motor trucks for a living. I didn't know what made a motor truck run. That wasn't all: I didn't want to know. I despised my job. I despised living in a cheap furnished room on West Fifty-sixth Street—a room infested with cockroaches. I still remember that I had a bunch of neckties hanging on the walls, and when I reached out every morning to get a fresh necktie, the cockroaches scattered in all directions. I despised having to eat in cheap, dirty restaurants that were also probably infested with cockroaches.

I came home to my lonely room each night with a sick headache—a headache bred and fed by disappointment, worry, bitterness, and rebellion. I was rebelling because the dreams I had nourished back in my college days had turned into nightmares. Was this life? Was this the vital adventure to which I had looked forward so eagerly? Was this all life would ever mean to me—working at a job I despised and with no hope for the future? I longed for leisure to read. I longed to write the books I had dreamed of writing back in my college days.

I knew I had everything to gain and nothing to lose by giving up the job I despised. I wasn't interested in making a lot of money, but I was interested in making a lot of living. In short, I had come to the Rubicon—to that moment of decision which faces most young people when they set out in life. So I made my decision, and that decision completely altered my future. It has made the rest of my life happy and rewarding beyond my most utopian aspiration.

My decision was this: I would give up the work I loathed, and since I had spent four years studying in the State Teachers College at Warrensburg, Missouri, preparing to teach, I would make my living teaching adult classes in night schools. Then I would have my days free to read books, prepare lectures, write novels and short stories. I wanted "to live to write and write to live."

—Dale Carnegie

Dale Carnegie never wrote the great American novel, but his remarkable success as a teacher, a businessman, and a writer of human-relations books has made him an inspiration to people around the world. He achieved all that by setting goals for himself, adjusting those goals as circumstances required, and trying never to lose sight of where he was headed next.

Mary Lou Retton was just a high-school sophomore from West Virginia, a state that had never once produced a world-class gymnast.

"I was a nobody," she says, "and I was number one in the state." She was a tiny fourteen-year-old, performing at a competition in Reno, Nevada. That's the day the great Bela

Karolyi, the Romanian gymnastics coach who had guided Nadia Comaneci to Olympic gold, walked up behind Mary Lou.

"He was the king of gymnastics," Retton recalls. "He came up to me. He tapped me on the shoulder. He's a big man—six-three or six-four. He came up to me and said, 'Mary Lou,' in that deep Romanian accent. 'You come to me, and I will make you Olympic champion.'"

The first thought that went racing through Retton's mind was, "Yeah, right. No way."

But of all the gymnasts in that Nevada arena, Bela Karolyi had noticed her. "So we sat down, and we talked," Retton remembers. "He talked with my parents and said, 'Listen, there's no guarantee that Mary Lou will even make the Olympic team, but I think she's got the material that it takes.'"

What a goal that was! Since early childhood she had harbored dreams about one day performing in the Olympics. But hearing the words come out of the great man's mouth—as far as Retton was concerned, that set the goal in stone.

"It was a very big risk for me," she says. "I was going to be moving away from my family and my friends, living with a family I had never met before, training with girls I didn't know. It pumped me up so much. I was scared. I didn't know what to expect. But I was excited too. This man wanted to train me. Little me, from Fairmont, West Virginia. I had been picked out."

And she wasn't about to let Karolyi down. It was two and a half years later that Mary Lou Retton, after a pair of perfect tens, won the Olympic gold medal in gymnastics for America—and with it a place in the hearts of people everywhere.

Goals give us something to shoot for. They keep our efforts focused. They allow us to measure our success.

So set goals—goals that are challenging but also realistic, goals that are clear and measurable, goals for the short term and goals for the long term.

When you reach one goal, take a second to pat yourself on the back. Then move on to the next goal, emboldened, strengthened, energized by what you've already achieved.

Eugene Lang, a New York City philanthropist, was making a graduation speech to a sixth-grade class at PS 121. This class had a group of children with absolutely no hope of ever going to college. In fact, there was very little hope that most of these children would even graduate from high school. But at the end of the graduation speech, Lang made a stunning offer. "For any of you who graduate from high school, I will ensure that funds are available for you to go to college," he said.

Of the forty-eight students in that sixth-grade class that day, forty-four graduated from high school and forty-two went to college. To put that into perspective, remember that forty percent of inner-city students never graduate from high school, let alone go to college.

That monetary offer alone wasn't enough to ensure such great success. Lang also made sure that the students got the support they needed along the way. They were monitored and counseled through their last six years of school. But that one challenging goal, clearly articulated and within the students' reach, gave them an opportunity to visualize a future they never thought was possible. And by visualizing it for themselves, they were able to make their dreams reality.

In the words of Harvey Mackay, the best-selling business author, "A goal is a dream with a deadline."

Howard Marguleas is the chairman of a produce company called Sun World, and he's one of California's new breed of growers. He got to be that way by setting and meeting goal after goal. For years Marguleas had watched as the agriculture business went up and down—fat times, lean times, as impossible to predict as they were to control. At least that's how everyone said the fruit-and-vegetable business worked.

But Marguleas had a goal: to develop new and unique kinds of produce that could withstand the shifts in the tides of consumer buying. "This business is really no different from real estate," Marguleas reasoned. "When the market's down, unless you have something very highly, uniquely different, you're in serious trouble. Same thing in agriculture. If you're just another producer of lettuce, carrots, or oranges, and you have nothing different from anyone else, you do well only if there's a short supply. If there's a large supply, you won't do well. And that's what we've tried to adjust to, to find the windows of opportunity that come with being different, a niche in the marketplace."

That's where the idea of a better pepper came from. Yes, a better pepper. If he could develop a pepper that was tastier than the peppers that other people grew, Marguleas assured himself, wouldn't the grocers of America want to stock it in good times and in bad?

So he did it, giving birth to the Le Rouge Royal pepper. "It's an elongated, three-lobe pepper," Marguleas says. "We were told, you know, 'You have to have a bell pepper, a square-shaped pepper, to sell.' But once we tasted this pepper—the color, the flavor, everything about it—we knew we had something. We knew that if we promoted it properly and advertised and merchandised it and put a name on it, we could get people to eat it. And once they ate it, they were going to continue to buy it."

What all this taught Marguleas is, "Never cease to pursue the opportunity to seek something different. Don't be satisfied with what you're doing. Always try to seek a way and a method to improve upon what you're doing, even if it's considered contrary to the traditions of an industry."

Those who fail to establish independent goals for themselves become, in Marguleas's word, the "me-toos" of the world. The me-toos, the people who follow but don't lead, do fine when times are good. But when times get tough, they inevitably get left behind.

Marguleas had his finger on something there. People who set goals—challenging goals, but goals that are also achievable—are the ones with solid grips on their futures, the ones who end up accomplishing extraordinary things.

Reebok International, Ltd., the athletic-shoe company, set a major corporate goal for itself: get Shaquille O'Neal. The Orlando Magic star wasn't going to come easy. Lots of major companies were eager to hire him as their spokesman.

"It was a question of convincing him that we had the best commitment to him, that we were willing to do something to create for him a program that the next guy couldn't do," says Paul Fireman, Reebok's chairman.

The whole company geared up. "We created an ad campaign before he was here. We created it for him exclusively. We spent money to create it, and we really put our effort in. We were just absolutely committed to getting him. We took a gamble. We took a risk. We spent the money, the time, and the commitment." Sometimes that's what setting goals is all about.

"It would have been a major confrontation emotionally if we had lost," Fireman said. "If we didn't go so far to get him here, we wouldn't have had the loss emotionally. But we wouldn't have had the player, either."

Goals aren't important only for companies. They're the building blocks that successful careers are made of.

Jack Gallagher worked in the family tire business, where he had held just about every job—accounting, bookkeeping, manufacturing, and sales. All that experience in the tire business taught him one thing for sure: he didn't want to work in the tire business.

One day Gallagher ran into a high-school friend who was working as an assistant administrator at a local hospital. "That's what I'd like to do," Gallagher told himself. "I'd love to help people. I'd love to have a big business, and I'd love to lead a group for the right things." There were several giant hurdles between Jack Gallagher and a hospital administrator's job—a graduate degree in hospital administration, for one thing, and a job at a hospital, for another.

But Gallagher had his goal, and he got started jumping the hurdles right away.

He talked his way into Yale. He won a stipend from the Kellogg Foundation. He got a loan from a local bank. He worked nights in the business office of North Shore University Hospital. And after he got the graduate degree, he applied for an administrative residency at North Shore.

"I interviewed with Jack Hausman, the chairman of the hospital's board," Gallagher recalls. "I must have spent three minutes with him, and I sold him in three minutes. He asked me a funny question. He knew I was married and had three kids. He said, 'How are you going to afford it?' They paid thirty-nine hundred for a resident then."

Gallagher recalls how he responded: "Look, Mr. Hausman, I thought it out a long time before I came to see you here. I had to have everything set so I could live during this residency and move into an administrative role after that."

He had a goal. He planned every detail. He worked tirelessly toward them. He's North Shore's CEO today.

Singer-songwriter Neil Sedaka, whose pop-music career has spanned more than three decades, learned to set goals when he was just a kid. Sedaka grew up in a rough part of Brooklyn, and he was never one of the tough guys. His earliest goal was a perfectly understandable one: to be liked and thereby stay alive through high school.

"I wasn't a fighter," Sedaka explained recently. "So I had to be liked. I always wanted to be liked. You know how it is. You're always afraid of getting into a fight." Anyway, young Neil came up with what turned out to be an ingenious method of achieving his personal goal—music.

"There was a sweetshop near Lincoln High School, and there was a jukebox in the back," he recalled. "All the tough kids, the leather-set kids, would hang out there, and they would listen to Elvis and Fats Domino. This was the beginning of rock and roll. So I wrote a rock-and-roll song, and I sang it, and then I was like a hero with those leather-set kids. They even let me into their part of the sweetshop."

The point here isn't whether Sedaka should have cared about acceptance from the tough kids. These things can seem awfully important in the high-school years. But he knew instinctively how to reach these other people—and how to achieve what was important to him at the time. For Sedaka, that high-school goal turned into a lifelong career, and this early success gave him the confidence to shoot for the stars in the future.

Much the same process unfolded in the early life of Arthur Ashe, the late tennis champion. Almost single-handedly, Ashe broke down the color barrier in professional tennis, a game that until he came along had been almost exclusively white. In his later years, Ashe fought a valiant battle against the AIDS virus, raising consciousness about the disease on ghetto street corners and in townhouse drawing rooms. His was a life of setting and reaching goals. For Ashe it started when he was a youngster on a tennis court. That's where he learned about achievement, one goal at a time.

"Breaking through that barrier, where you have set a goal and you achieve that goal, it sort of codifies whatever budding self-confidence you might have had," Ashe said in an interview for this book just before his death.

That's how Ashe operated until the day he died. He'd set a goal and when he'd met that goal, he'd set another one. Why? "The self-confidence itself, I think, transforms the individual," he explained. "It also spills over into other areas of life. Not only do you feel confident in whatever you are expert at, but you probably feel generally self-confident that you can do some other things as well, applying the same principles maybe to another task or to another set of goals."

The goals must be realistic, and they must be attainable. Don't make the mistake of thinking you should, or can, accomplish everything today. Maybe you can't reach the moon this year, so plan a shorter trip. Set an interim goal.

Following that incremental approach, Ashe put himself on the big-time tennis map. "My early coaches," explained Ashe, "set out definite goals which I bought into. The goals were not necessarily winning tennis tournaments. The goals were just things that we saw as difficult, that would require some hard work and some planning. And there was sort of an implied reward out there if I achieved those goals. Again, the goal wasn't necessarily winning this tournament or that tournament. And so incrementally, before I knew it, after I attained these mini goals along the way, all of a sudden, 'Hey, I'm close to the big prize here.'"

That's how Ashe always approached tough tennis matches. "In a tournament, you'd want to get to the quarterfinals. Or in a match, you would want to not miss a certain number of backhand passing shots. Or maybe you'd want to improve your stamina to a point where you're not going to get tired when the weather is too hot. Those are the sorts of goals that help take your general focus off that long-range, elusive goal—the goal of being number one or winning the whole tournament."

Most big challenges are best faced with a series of interim goals. That's a far more encouraging process—far more motivating too.

Dr. James D. Watson, the director of the Cold Spring Harbor Laboratory, has been locked in a lifelong struggle to find the cure for cancer. Is that his only goal? Of course not. That would be too discouraging for anyone to bear. Watson has laid out a series of incremental goals for himself and his laboratory colleagues, goals they are meeting every year on the road to the ultimate cure.

"There are so many different cancers," explains Watson, who won a Nobel prize for discovering the structure of DNA. "We're going to cure some of them. Hopefully, we'll cure more of them.

"But you've got to pick interim goals," he says. "The goal is not to kill colon cancer tomorrow. It's to understand the disease. And there are many different steps. No one wants to be led into defeat. You get your happiness one small goal at a time."

That's the way it works. Set little goals. Meet them. Set new, slightly larger goals. Meet them. Succeed.

Long before Lou Holtz became Notre Dame's head football coach, he wanted nothing more than to play the game himself. But when he went out for his high-school team, he weighed just 115 pounds.

Holtz knew this was far too small. Still, he desperately wanted to play, so he came up with a plan. He memorized all eleven positions on the team. That way, if any player got hurt, he was immediately prepared to rush onto the field. It gave him eleven chances instead of one.

"It's the same way in business today," says writer Harvey

Mackay. "If you're working out here in the office, volunteer to learn the phone system. Volunteer to know what's going on in computers. If you're in sales, you want to know about computers." That way, when opportunities appear, you'll have a much greater chance of seizing them. Set goals that make you more valuable to your team—as Lou Holtz did—or to your company.

The idea is to set goals and then strive to meet them. Sometimes you'll succeed on schedule, sometimes things will take longer to achieve than you thought, and sometimes you won't attain what you thought you would. Some things just aren't meant to be. The point is to keep planning and plugging away. You'll get there, just watch.

As Scalamandré Silks' Adriana Bitter says: "Maybe we set our goals too high sometimes and we don't always reach the top end, but we certainly can start climbing that ladder."

Without specific goals it's far too easy just to drift, never really taking charge of your life. Time gets wasted because nothing has a sense of urgency. There's no deadline. Nothing has to be done *today*. It's possible to put off anything indefinitely. Goals are what can give us direction and keep us focused.

David Luther of Corning is acutely aware of this modern propensity toward aimlessness. He worries about how it might affect his own children at home. So he's constantly talking to them about goals.

"Sometimes," he reminds them, "we get caught up in things." Easy to say, of course, but how to avoid this pitfall? "The point," according to Luther, "is to know yourself. Think what it is that you know and want to do. Forget the money, for a moment anyway. When you get to be the age of your parents, what is it you want to be able to point to that met your expectation, that made a difference?"

How are intelligent goals created? Mostly they just take a little thought, but there are some useful techniques for getting the mind focused on the task. You might try asking yourself the same questions Luther urges his children to ask. "Stand back and say, 'What is it I really want to be? What kind of life do I really want to lead? Am I heading in the right direction now?'" That advice makes sense no matter how far along you are in your career.

Once you establish what your goals are, prioritize them. Not everything can be done at once, so you've got to ask yourself, Which comes first? What goal is most important to me now? Then try organizing your time and energy to reflect those priorities. This, often, is the most challenging part.

To prioritize his goals, Ted Owen, publisher of the *San Diego Business Journal*, follows the advice he got from a psychologist friend. "He told me to take a piece of paper and draw a line down the center. On the left, put any number you want. I put ten. Put the top ten things that you want to accomplish in your life before you retire at whatever age that is, one hundred or sixty or fifty.

"Put down those ten things. So you want to have a good retirement program. You want to have a nice home. You want to have a happy marriage. You want to have good health. Whatever those ten are. Then over here on the other side, you take those ten and prioritize them. One of those ten becomes number one, and so on."

Simplistic? Maybe. But helpful too. Through this process, Owen discovered some things about himself he never knew. "I found out that a job, a well-paying, steady job, a job that makes me feel good, was about number seven." Once you identify your own number one, two, three, and seven, creating well-crafted goals becomes a whole lot easier.

It's fine if, over the years, those goals develop and change. "Before I was married, I would come in on the weekends just to read the newspaper here," says Dr. Ronald Evans, a research professor at the Salk Institute for Biological Studies. "I had nothing else to do. I loved being in labs. It was sort of a home away from home. Research is addicting," he observes. "It's incredibly challenging and pushes your intellectual limits. You make discoveries, and there's nothing like it."

But life changes, pressures change, and goals should be evaluated too. "With a family now," Evans goes on, "it's been very difficult to change my habits, but I have. You just have to say you can't do everything."

Corporations need goals as much as individuals do, and the same basic rules apply when companies begin defining theirs: make them clear, keep them basic, and don't set too many at once.

The huge Motorola corporation was run in one recent year with just three specific goals, expressed in precise, mathematical terms: to "continue 10-X improvement" every two years, to "get the voice of" the customer, to "cut business-process cycle time by factor 10" in five years.

Don't worry about what this language means. It may or may not apply at your company. What's important here is that the company has its goals. These goals are clearly understood within the company. The goals are challenging but attainable. Progress is easily measurable. And if these goals are achieved, the company will have done extraordinarily well.

Those three specific goals provide enough vision to run an entire company. Imagine what three equally clear, equally realistic goals can do for one person's life.

SET GOALS THAT ARE CLEAR, CHALLENGING, AND OBTAINABLE.

7

THE BASIC ATTITUDE THAT BRINGS WEALTH AND PEACE OF MIND

Napoleon Hill

A life of wealth enjoyed by a mind at peace comes most often to men who maintain a positive mental attitude. With definiteness of purpose you add great positive power to your own mental attitude, and you can use definite motives to sustain the actions which propel you toward your goal. At the same time you can set up spiritual guardians to keep your attitudes at a high "Yes" level, avoid conflicts of motive, tune-in on other positive minds.

The computers which are beginning to manage our world are complicated devices. Most of them, however, have a very simple basic principle: they say Yes or No. They either open a kind of electrical gate or they keep it closed, and by multiplying this process they can assimilate and select all kinds of information.

The mind of man is far more wonderful than any machine. Within it, however, there seems to be a kind of Yes-No valve at the focal point of thinking. It is as though your awareness of a circumstance of life—sent to your brain by your sight, hearing and other senses—presents itself at the Yes-No point to be processed. A person who maintains a positive attitude will find every possible Yes in that circumstance and make it part of his life. A person who maintains a negative mental attitude will lean toward the No side, miss much that is good, live with much that is painful and damaging.

Nothing but a mental attitude? Nothing but a mental attitude, but it is right there that your success or your failure, your peace of mind or your nervous tension, your tendency toward good health or your tendency toward illness begins.

Fortunately it is possible for anyone to make the change from negativism to positivism, and thus basically condition his brain to bring all that is good in life. Moreover, there are certain "control levers" which the Creator makes available to us, and it is easy to see how successful people use these levers, once you know what they are.

I shall give you some here and some in other chapters so as to reinforce your memory. Now and then you will find repetition of names, facts and methods in this book, always with a view toward helping you remember.

Control your mental attitude with definiteness of purpose. Emerson said: "The world makes way for a man who knows where he is going."

Think what it means to know where you are going! Automatically you rid yourself of all kinds of fears and doubts which may have crept into the making-up-your-mind process. Your purpose is definite and—presto!—all the limitless forces of your mind focus upon that purpose and no other. Knowing your purpose, you cannot be led astray by circumstances or words which have nothing to do with your purpose. Where, before, a day's work may have contained a good deal of wasted motion, now your efforts are lined up so that each mental or physical motion helps every other motion.

You can see the connection with building wealth, for work done well is a basic wealth-builder. Now see the connection with peace of mind. A man who works wholeheartedly at his job is not concerned with such matters as finding fault with others, disturbing his conscience by cutting corners in his work, watching the clock and so forth. Nor will he be discouraged by any obstacles which may crop up; his positive and focused mental attitude keeps him in a prime position to handle problems and overcome them.

EFFICIENCY AND POSITIVITY

Is this a secret of "genius"? I have mentioned that many eminently successful men do not possess any greater intelligence than most other men possess. Yet their achievements are such that we may say that these men have "genius." Surely it is the positive mental attitude of these men which makes their brain-power, not greater, but more efficient and more available than most others'. When I spoke to such men as Henry Ford, Andrew Carnegie and Thomas A. Edison, I spoke with minds free of any fear or doubt that they could do anything they wished to do.

I know that Andrew Carnegie was well aware of the need for a positive mental attitude. Before he undertook to back me in my success, he really put me "on the spot" as to my mental attitude.

Looking at me shrewdly across his desk, that canny Scot said: "We've talked a long time and I have shown you the greatest opportunity a young man ever had to become famous, rich and useful. Now—if I choose you out of the two hundred and forty other applicants for this job—if I introduce you to the outstandingly successful men in America—if I help you get their collaboration in finding out the true philosophy of success—will you devote twenty years to the job, earning your own living as you go along? We have had sufficient discussion. I want your answer—yes or no."

I began to think of all the obstacles that would stand in my way. I began to think of all the hurdles I would have to jump. I began to think of all the time I would have to spend, and the big job of writing, and the problem of earning my living all that while—and so forth.

I spent twenty-nine seconds struggling with a negative mental attitude which, had it overcome me, would have affected me negatively ever after.

How do I know I took just twenty-nine seconds? Because, when I found the positive mental attitude which I had lost temporarily, and said "Yes!"—Mr. Carnegie showed me the stopwatch he had been holding beneath his desk. He had given me just one minute in which to show my positive state of mind otherwise, he felt, he would not have been able to depend on it. I had beaten the deadline by just thirty-one seconds, and thereby embraced an opportunity that was destined to change and improve the lives of millions of people, including my own.

A positive mind tunes in on other positive minds. Once I had accepted that great task and had set my mind confidently toward it, I found that my imagined obstacles simply melted away. Of course my positive mental attitude helped me not only in finding out the success secrets of some five hundred of America's wealthiest men, but also in making considerably more than a mere living. Am I a genius? I must say I have positive evidence I am not!

In meeting many men I discovered a very valuable fact: a positive mind automatically obtains benefit from other positive minds.

Are you aware of the general principle of radio broadcasting? It is this: when electrical vibrations of rapid frequency are impressed upon a wire, those vibrations leap into space. Another wire far away—the receiving antenna—can pick them up, and thus a message or a picture is transmitted over thousands of miles, or millions of miles in space-age communication.

There are electrical currents in the brain. They give you a private broadcasting station through which you may send out any kind of thought vibrations you desire. Keep that station busy sending out thoughts of a positive nature, thoughts which will benefit others, and you will find you can receive kindred thought vibrations from other minds whose attitude is tuned to yours.

When I visited such successful men as those I have mentioned, and many others such as John Wanamaker, Frank A. Vanderlip, Edward Bok and Woodrow Wilson, both they and I felt the attunement of mind to mind. Otherwise I surely would have met with opposition when I asked those top-ranking men to give me of their time and experience. Not only did such men spend hours talking to me, but also they served as my teachers and guides for year after year, and charged me nothing.

Believe in what you are doing, and you too will see the great effect of your belief upon those whom you may request to help you. Doubt yourself and the No part of your mind takes over and draws defeat instead of victory.

This barely sketches in the all-pervasive power of a positive mental attitude. Let us look at some of the other "control levers" which combine with a positive mental attitude to give you wealth and peace of mind for an entire, victorious lifetime.

THE NINE MAJOR MOTIVES

It is not for nothing that court trials often concern themselves with questions of motive. Everything you do is the result of one or more motives. In various combinations we use nine basic motives. The seven positive motives are:

1. The emotion of LOVE
2. The emotion of SEX
3. The desire for MATERIAL GAIN
4. The desire for SELF-PRESERVATION
5. The desire for FREEDOM OF BODY AND MIND
6. The desire for SELF-EXPRESSION
7. The desire for PERPETUATION OF LIFE AFTER DEATH

The two negative emotions are:

1. The emotion of ANGER AND REVENGE
2. The emotion of FEAR

In those nine motives you can find the roots of everything you do or refrain from doing. Peace of mind is attained only by the exercise of the seven positive motives as a general pattern of life. Rarely if ever does a person who has peace of mind exercise the two negative motives or emotions. You cannot have peace of mind while you fear anything or anyone. You cannot have peace of mind while you entertain the kind of anger which brings you to a desire for revenge or a desire to injure another, no matter what the justification may seem to be.

THE PRICE OF PEACE OF MIND

Great men have no time to waste with a desire to injure others. If they did, they would not be great men. Great men are not immune to fear, but theirs is not the kind of fear that hangs on constantly and takes over all of life. Look to small, mean men to see lifelong patterns of fear and anger. Their minds are so filled with these negative influences that they cannot find the power to shape the circumstances they desire.

Recently I heard about a man, now seventy, who fifteen years ago lost all his money in a real estate venture. Taking the advice of a friend, he had borrowed heavily in order to invest in vacant swampland on the assumption that in a couple of years the land would be in great demand for building lots. This did not transpire, the man's notes became due, and he had to see his retail shoe business sold out from under him.

The friend who had badly advised him also had lost money. Nevertheless this man became filled with hatred toward his friend and said he would get even "if it's the last thing I do." It nearly was. Five years of hatred left him incapable even of doing business. Meanwhile the friend prospered and seemed far out of reach of any puny revenge. The man who had lost his money at length lost the balance wheel of his mind and had to spend six months in a quiet place in the country surrounded by a high wall.

In his last month of confinement, however, he was sufficiently recovered to listen to an adviser who pointed out to him that hatred and the desire for revenge had done him far more harm than had been done by his losing his money. He was persuaded to forgive the friend who had led him into the real estate deal. He even wrote to this man, telling of his change of heart.

When he went back into business it was with love of his fellow men and the determination to keep his mind filled with positive, constructive motives. Beginning at the age of sixty, he built a new career. Now, at seventy, he is fairly well off, and most of all he has peace of mind, the one form of wealth which is indispensable.

I myself have suffered from the effects of negative motives from time to time. When I went into hiding, as discussed in the last chapter, I acted at first upon a very wise motive of self-preservation. Soon, however, this turned into fear and with the fear came misery. Fortunately I saw in time what was happening to me. It cannot happen again.

You can call upon Ten Princes of Guidance to stand at the doors of your mind. You can make yourself aware of certain principles of personal guidance and guardianship; and to make these principles real and memorable, you can personalize them— see them as so many Princes in armor who stand at the doors of your mind. These Princes challenge every thought-vibration which seeks to enter. They keep your mind positive, effective and free of discord. I shall name my own Princes, a list which you may wish to modify to suit your own life-requirements.

The Prince of Peace of Mind. He stands at the very outer door and asks all callers if they come in peace to share my peace. If not, they are turned away.

The Prince of Hope and Faith. He admits only those influences which keep my mind alerted with belief in my mission in life.

The Prince of Love and Romance. He brings into my mind only those influences which keep love eternally fresh in my heart.

The Prince of Sound Physical Health. He knows the kind of mental influences which can destroy health, and admits only those states of mind which help the body maintain its vigor.

The Prince of Financial Security. When I desire him to stand on guard, he admits no thoughts save those which bring me worthy financial benefit.

The Prince of Overall Wisdom. He is charged with passing certain thoughts into my store of knowledge when he sees they will benefit me or help me benefit others.

The Prince of Patience. He keeps away all impulses to rush, to tackle jobs half-prepared, to be in any way impatient with the power of time.

The Prince of Normhill. "Normhill" is a very personal word I have created for my own use. Combining certain names, it means to me what it cannot mean to any other. Just so, create your own name for your own very personal Prince. This Prince stands guard along with all the others. The others from time to time may be relieved of duty; for instance, one hardly may wish continually to keep out all thoughts except those which have to do with financial security. Your special personal Prince is always there, representing all the special personal influences in your life. Normhill is my ambassador-at-large who performs services not assigned to the other members of my invisible family of guides.

When you have made yourself well aware of your corps of spiritual Princes, they serve to rally all your forces to solve any problem or to set up special lines of defense.

Sometimes I find myself talking to someone whose antagonistic attitude begins to invade my peace of mind. Very well—I send a special alert to the Prince of Peace of Mind. Immediately he takes charge of the ramparts with doubled strength, and I am calm and in control of my own mind once more.

Or, let us say, I feel some physical ache or pain. I call upon the Prince of Sound Physical Health to look into the cause, and I get good results. I believe I have received benefits of healing which are beyond the power of ordinary medical science to explain.

My Princes of Guidance receive a certain compensation for their services. Their "pay" is my eternal gratitude. Daily I express this gratitude, first to each of the Princes individually, then to all of them in their mighty group. You will find this expression of gratitude of great help in keeping your mind alerted to its own powers. I know that if I ever neglect it, I feel a neglect on the part of my Princes. When, once again, I make myself aware every day that I have great spiritual forces at my command—there they are once more, as strong as ever.

Don't let the motive of material gain conflict with the motive of freedom. Freedom of body is easy to see and understand; but freedom of mind is a subtle matter. Fear and anger put the mind behind bars. Guilt wraps the mind in chains. To add a bit of levity to a serious matter: Once there was a man who was encouraged to know himself. Immediately he handcuffed himself to his bed, so he would not get up and rifle his own pockets during the night.

All too often the motive of material gain—excellent in itself—conflicts with the excellent motive of freedom of body and mind because in gaining what is material we give up freedom of mind; we load the mind with guilt and fear because we do not act honestly.

In addition, one who makes his money through taking dishonest advantage of his fellow men has cheated himself of the genuine joy which comes with honest success. When you obey the rules of a game, and win, you have done something for your soul. When you cheat and win, you only call it winning, but you have really lost instead.

I believe I was fortunate in starting my career very early

in life, so that I learned life's lessons quite early. Let me tell you of an experience I had while I was holding my first job. I was just out of business college and I was inexperienced in the ways of life and the character of men.

My employer owned a number of banks. He had placed his son as a cashier of one of his banks, in a distant town. One night a hotel manager in that town telephoned me, saying my employer's son was in serious difficulty. He had not been able to reach my employer. Immediately, I boarded the train and arrived in the town early the next morning.

When I went to the bank I found the door closed but unlocked. Inside, I discovered that the vault had been left open and beautiful green currency was scattered all over the teller's counter.

I closed the door and picked up the telephone. I managed to get my employer on the phone and told him why I had gone to that town and what I had found on my arrival. In great distress, he said: "Go ahead and count the money. Balance the books. Draw a draft on me for whatever shortage there may be."

I settled down to counting the money. To my great surprise, not a cent was missing.

I sat there looking at those piles of greenbacks. My youth had been tragic, turbulent and poor. My present state was one of bare solvency. I sat there looking at nearly $50,000 in cash, knowing that I could put at least half of it into my pocket and nobody would be the wiser. My employer's son showed obvious signs of mental instability. Everyone would assume he had taken the money. He even had acted as though he had filled his own pockets—and I was the only one who knew he had not.

The motive of material gain nudged heavily at me. But the motive of freedom said: Don't do it. Or rather, it was "something" that kept me honest, for at that time I could not have named the major motives. Perhaps that "something" was the result of certain sessions I had had with my stepmother before I had left home, in which she had instilled into me the fact that I was in control of my own mind and that always I must live with myself.

I locked the money into the vault forthwith, then phoned my employer and told him there was no deficiency to make up; not a cent had been stolen. I walked out of that bank with a mind at peace, a mind that was free and joyously positive.

Forever after I have placed the motive of freedom ahead of the motive of material gain. I have succeeded in having all the money I need without ever hampering either my inward or outward freedom.

LIFE IS A MIRROR

This episode was one of several which led me straight to Andrew Carnegie and my realization of my goal in life. My employer was grateful for the way in which I had protected his son's reputation as best I could. He was responsible later for my entering Georgetown University Law School. This led through a chain of circumstances to my assignment to interview Mr. Carnegie. If I had yielded to the material gain motive that day in the bank, the Science of Personal Achievement might never have come into being.

Yes, as Emerson suggested, there is a silent partner in all our transactions, and woe is the lot of the man who tries to drive a sharp bargain with Life.

Life reflects your own thoughts back to you. Thoughts are things, a poet said, and truly they have an existence of their own, so that a curse comes back to curse you and a blessing comes back to bless you, reflected by the mighty mirror of life. Another poet said: "I am the master of my fate, I am the captain of my soul." This too is true, and the two truths harmonize. Send out positive thoughts from a positively oriented soul and the world will reflect back greater and greater positive influences to help you.

Turn back and read the list of nine basic motives. Concentrate on the seven positive motives. Remember it is possible for these motives to come into conflict, as we have seen; but by and large they drive one way, and with a positive mental attitude they take you the way you want to go. We shall not say farewell to the motives till we are finished with this book; but let us now pay our respects briefly.

Love has limitless scope. Handle it in a spirit of reverence, for it is tuned to the Eternal. Give freely of it and you will attract as much as or more than you give; stop giving love and you stop receiving. With no other emotion or motive or desire is the mirror of life so very evident.

Sex is the great creative force of the universe. On its highest plane it merges with love; but love can exist without being sexual. The mighty power of sex can be transmuted into action for the achievement of profound purpose, and so important is this matter that later on we shall devote an entire chapter to it. On the other hand, sex may be debauched and misused, and it is in this guise that it brings grief and trouble to mankind and gives itself an underserved bad reputation.

Self-preservation can become a negative force when one seeks it without regard to the rights of other people. It is instilled by Nature to help us stay alive. Even so, the human being assumes the prerogative of rising above it. When a ship is sinking it is women and children first, and there are many parallel instances which call forth a nobility in human nature.

Self-expression is part of finding one's self. It is part of one's freedom to be one's self. Thus it is positive, constructive and infinitely valuable. Only make sure that your own means of self-expression do not demean or damage others.

Perpetuation of life after death belongs among the earliest beliefs and motives of mankind. It should be bounded by common sense and a true understanding of one's relationship to that change known as death. When wrapped in superstition and fear, this motive leads only to wretchedness. It can turn life into a preparation for death and hamper an entire civilization.

THE SUREST WAY OF FINDING PEACE OF MIND

The surest way of finding peace of mind is that which helps the greatest number of others to find it.

Let this be your guide to your use of the great motivating forces; then you will know you are using them correctly, not corrupting them.

Is there peace of mind in prayer? There can be. There should be. But note how many people go to prayer only in the hour of a misfortune, when the motive of fear dominates their minds. The approach must be negative in that case, and so, in terms of peace of mind, the results must be negative as well.

Prayers which bring peace of mind proceed from a mind which gives forth a confident message even though that mind may be afflicted with problems and sorrow. Prayers which free great forces to solve problems are born in minds which know that the problems can be solved once the forces are found—and have perfect confidence in the existence of those forces.

Along with many others I see evidence of an Intelligence beyond man's. I believe that the positively conditioned mind may at times tune in on that Intelligence. Yet mind-conditioning through prayer or resolution is something an individual must accomplish for himself. When the Creator made man free to seek his own destiny, and choose between good and evil, he gave man this prerogative as well. Every great accomplishment of any man at any time first had to exist as a thought before it could exist as reality.

Have you recognized the Supreme Secret?

8

CONQUERING BURNOUT AND STRESS

Roger Fritz

"Expect trouble as an inevitable part of life and when it comes, hold your head high, look it squarely in the eye and say, 'I will be bigger than you. You cannot defeat me.'"

—Ann Landers

Every profession inherently carries its own dose of stress. In fact, a certain level of stress is vital to keep engagement alive; it injects a sense of challenge that prevents monotony from settling in. However, it's the tipping point where stress transforms into distress that issues arise. This transition often manifests through behavioral shifts. Individuals known for their unwavering patience might suddenly exhibit signs of impatience. Normally composed individuals might display visible tension. Employees, once highly cooperative, might exhibit rebellious tendencies. Others may endure physical manifestations, expressing difficulty falling asleep or maintaining a restful night's sleep. Even after a seemingly good rest, they might persistently battle fatigue, experiencing stomach discomfort, a racing heart, or frequent headaches.

While physical rest can alleviate bodily fatigue, mental

fatigue often persists in the workplace. This mental drain can be particularly pronounced in roles heavily reliant on computer work. Encouraging physical exercise emerges as a viable remedy. Encourage those in computer-centric roles to engage in physical activities, perhaps suggesting a lunchtime stroll, swimming, jogging, or participation in a sport post-work hours. Numerous companies are now providing exercise facilities where employees can utilize stationary bikes or weight machines during their lunch breaks. Those who adhere to a consistent exercise routine tend to exhibit lower susceptibility to mental exhaustion.

By promoting physical activity as a means to counter mental fatigue, workplaces are acknowledging the interconnectedness of physical and mental well-being. Incorporating such practices not only fosters a healthier workforce but also underscores the significance of holistic wellness in combating workplace stress.

> "You cannot tailor-make the situations in life, but you can tailor-make the attitudes to fit those situations before they arise."
>
> —Zig Ziglar

BURNOUT

Unlike light bulbs, people don't burn out abruptly like a sudden flicker in brightness followed by an abrupt outage. Human burnout is a gradual, often imperceptible process. While some instances may result in physical breakdowns like heart attacks or ulcers, the majority are primarily psychological. The signs of burnout are subtle yet pervasive. Individuals slowly lose their zest, vitality, and drive, which manifests in various ways. They find themselves disliking their job, experiencing friction with colleagues, harboring distrust toward team leaders, and harboring a pervasive sense of dread every morning as they contemplate heading to work.

Excessive stress is a prominent trigger for burnout, but it's not the sole culprit. Frustration stemming from unfulfilled promises, overlooked expected promotions or salary increments, or the relentless pressure of making critical decisions leading to potential catastrophic outcomes can all fuel burnout. Furthermore, extended work hours or unfulfilling roles are additional contributors. Those equipped with a positive mindset often navigate these challenges more adeptly.

Identifying burnout is relatively more straightforward than finding a cure. Its markers include diminished assertiveness, a tolerance for mediocrity, waning motivation to enhance performance, declining productivity, and deteriorating relationships. Implementing these suggestions serves as a proactive strategy to halt the descent into a state of stagnation and disillusionment.

TEST YOUR STRESS LEVEL

Work on this stress assessment to gauge the proximity of serious stress-related issues in your life. Take a moment to delve into these queries and assign your responses in the designated box. Employ "SA" for Strongly Affirmative, "A" for Affirmative, "N" for Negative, and "SN" for Strongly Negative.

1. _______ Are you frequently fatigued throughout the day, lacking energy?
2. _______ Do you find yourself less vocal or participative in business meetings compared to your previous engagement level?

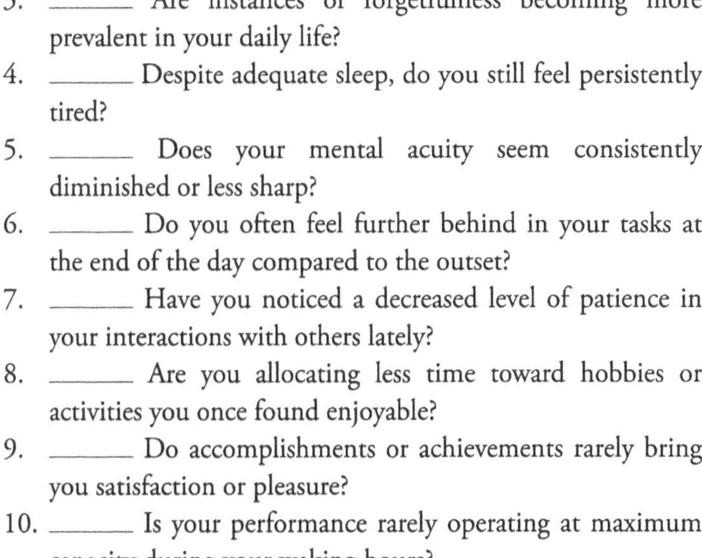

3. _______ Are instances of forgetfulness becoming more prevalent in your daily life?

4. _______ Despite adequate sleep, do you still feel persistently tired?

5. _______ Does your mental acuity seem consistently diminished or less sharp?

6. _______ Do you often feel further behind in your tasks at the end of the day compared to the outset?

7. _______ Have you noticed a decreased level of patience in your interactions with others lately?

8. _______ Are you allocating less time toward hobbies or activities you once found enjoyable?

9. _______ Do accomplishments or achievements rarely bring you satisfaction or pleasure?

10. _______ Is your performance rarely operating at maximum capacity during your waking hours?

Award yourself ten points for a Strongly Affirmative (SA) response, seven points for an Affirmative (A) answer, three points for a Negative (N) reply, and zero points for a Strongly Negative (SN) response.

Now, as you evaluate your cumulative score, consider the following ranges: A score between zero to 15 signifies a state of either complete inactivity or a well-organized life; a range of 16 to 50 indicates a lower likelihood of experiencing burnout; a score from 51 to 80 suggests a precarious position where burnout could be looming; and a score of 86 to 100 signifies an elevated risk, suggesting you might be teetering on the brink as a walking stress bomb. This assessment serves as a valuable tool to help recognize and potentially address burgeoning stress-related concerns in your life.

MANAGING STRESS

Effectively managing job-related stress requires proactive measures to mitigate its impact. While some physicians might advocate for tranquilizers or other medications, self-management of stress can be achieved through the following practices:

1. Prioritize your well-being by maintaining a healthy lifestyle. Pay attention to your diet and commit to a consistent exercise regimen to keep yourself in optimal shape.
2. Embrace relaxation techniques by engaging in structured relaxation exercises. Dedicate time for solitude to unwind and recharge.
3. Foster self-respect and nurture high self-esteem. Individuals with a robust sense of self-worth are often more resilient to external pressures.
4. Acknowledge that you cannot always please everyone, underlining the importance of setting realistic boundaries.
5. Cultivate a thirst for continuous learning. Embracing ongoing learning experiences keeps your mind alert, adaptable, and invigorated.
6. Establish a reliable support network. Surround yourself with friends and family who can provide support during challenging times.
7. Assess and accept commitments that truly align with your priorities. Politely decline tasks that may excessively drain your time and energy.
8. Foster creativity in your approach to tasks. Innovate by revisiting how you handle routine responsibilities and develop fresh, creative methods to tackle new challenges, reducing their stress-inducing impact.

9. Embrace change as an avenue for new opportunities rather than perceiving it as a threat.
10. Harness the power of positive thinking. Replace negative thought patterns with positive mental images, leveraging the proven benefits of optimistic perspectives.
11. Reassess leisure activities that add to your tension. If a hobby or leisure pursuit, such as competitive sports or high-stakes games like Tournament Bridge, exacerbates stress, consider replacing it with a genuinely relaxing alternative.
12. Grant yourself permission to lead a balanced life. Delight in activities with loved ones without feeling guilty for momentarily disengaging from work-related thoughts.

By adopting these strategies, you can proactively manage stress, fostering a more harmonious balance between professional obligations and personal well-being.

> "Adopting the right attitude can convert a negative stress into a positive one."
>
> —Hans Selye

COPING WITH BURNOUT

Achieving recovery from burnout necessitates a candid examination of fundamental issues that often contribute to this state:

1. Conflicting objectives: When the aspirations of the organization and your own ambitions diverge, a sense of misalignment emerges, creating a perception that

avenues for professional advancement and alignment are severely limited.

2. Monotonous and uninspiring tasks: An excess of routine work without room for exploration or intellectual challenge fosters a stagnant environment dominated by repetitive tasks.

3. Insufficient responsibility and influence: A scarcity of fresh challenges or an absence of opportunities to assume greater authority can contribute to a sense of stagnation and dissatisfaction.

4. Shifting personal priorities: Emerging familial needs or unexpected health concerns may alter the landscape, temporarily shifting the focus from career advancement to other pressing personal obligations.

5. Evolving educational or technical demands: Unforeseen educational or technical prerequisites can jeopardize the trajectory of high achievers unless these demands are anticipated and adequate time is allocated for their fulfillment.

6. Undervaluation despite significant effort: Instances where consistent dedication and tackling challenging tasks don't translate into commensurate recognition, praise, compensation, or promotion.

In such scenarios, taking proactive steps becomes pivotal:

1. Documenting incidents and experiences that highlight the mismatch between effort and acknowledgment.

2. Engaging in introspection, reevaluating personal goals, and aligning them with professional pursuits.

3. Initiating a meeting with relevant stakeholders to address and discuss concerns surrounding the perceived lack of acknowledgment. Proactively taking charge of

this conversation can potentially catalyze personal and professional growth, rather than passively waiting for external initiatives.

RELIEVING STRESS AT THE OFFICE

Alleviating stress in the office is a deeply personal journey as different approaches resonate uniquely with individuals. What proves effective for one might not necessarily yield the same results for another. However, there exist several strategies that can significantly contribute to a more balanced workday:

Taking a Timeout

Charley, when feeling the weight of undue pressure, implements a brief respite strategy. Stepping away from his desk, donning his coat, and exiting the building, he takes a short ten-minute walk around the block or the parking lot. This breather helps renew his vigor and grants him a refreshed perspective.

Similarly, Esther, situated in the downtown area, chooses to escape the stress by temporarily leaving the building. Her reprieve involves a calming session of window shopping in a nearby mall.

Contrarily, Stan, restricted by a boss who disapproves of leaving during work hours, opts for a change of environment within the building. By engaging in errands in different departments, he effectively redirects his mind and eases the mounting tension.

Incorporating Exercise

While doing jumping jacks might not be ideal in a room full of colleagues, subtle exercises like controlled breathing can be discreetly performed. Inhaling deeply through the nose and exhaling slowly through the mouth for several repetitions offers a calming effect, inducing relaxation throughout the body.

Ted, benefiting from a well-equipped company gym, utilizes a short stint on a stationary bike during high-stress moments, effectively alleviating tension without breaking a sweat.

Task Rotation

When pressure surges on a particular project, shifting focus to another task for a brief interval can provide respite. Heather, overwhelmed by an impending deadline, recognized her dwindling concentration. She temporarily set aside the pressing project, diverting her attention to a different assignment for half an hour. Returning to her primary task, her mind had cleared, allowing for a renewed approach.

Seeking Companionship

For some, confiding in a friend serves as a potent stress-relief mechanism. Peter opts to discuss his stress with a close friend, acknowledging that while he doesn't expect a solution, verbalizing his thoughts to someone else helps clarify his perspective. Furthermore, casual conversation often alleviates tension in mere moments.

Find Your Own Solution

When it comes to relieving tension, a myriad of approaches can prove effective. Take, for instance, the story of an individual who, when overwhelmed with stress, retreats to the confines of his car, meticulously closing the windows before releasing a visceral scream—a liberating act of release.

In a separate scenario, Dierdre, fortunate enough to possess a private office, found solace in the tranquil practice of yoga, dedicating a precious few minutes to untangling the knots of stress that accumulate throughout the day.

Then there's Jim, whose haven lies not in physical proximity but in the recesses of his mind. He mentally transports himself to the serene stream nestled near his summer abode, immersing his senses in the symphony of water cascading over the smooth, sun-kissed rocks—a mental oasis of peace.

For others, the path to tranquility unfolds through meditation or devout prayer, harnessing the power of mindfulness or spiritual connection to alleviate the burdens of workplace stress.

Each of these approaches, whether discovered through personal experimentation or embraced from existing practices, serves as a testament to the diverse arsenal available for stress reduction in the workplace. The key lies in uncovering a method that resonates with you, one that speaks to your unique needs and offers a personalized avenue to navigate the pressures of professional life.

> "Holding on to anger is like grasping a hot coal with the intent of throwing it at someone else—you are the one who gets burned."
>
> —Buddha

USING YOUR POSITIVE ATTITUDE TO HELP OTHERS

Your pivotal role in rejuvenating a burnt-out member of your team cannot be overstated. Your own positive attitude serves as a beacon of hope, illuminating the path to their recovery through a series of transformative actions:

Firstly, displaying unwavering support is paramount. Engage in sincere conversations, fostering an environment where concerns are not only welcomed but actively addressed. Facilitate necessary adjustments, showcasing genuine interest in their well-being.

Consider the potential for a metamorphosis in job functions. Altering tasks or transitioning to a different team can invigorate their professional landscape, injecting freshness and offering novel avenues for rejuvenation.

Offering opportunities for skill acquisition is a dual-edged solution. Not only does it redirect focus towards learning, but it also augments their value within the company, fostering a sense of growth and accomplishment.

Should these interventions falter to yield progress, the prudent step is to advocate for professional counseling. This proactive approach can provide specialized guidance and support, acknowledging the complexity of the situation and offering targeted assistance.

Understanding your behavioral inclinations is merely the first step. Recognizing these tendencies acts as a clarion call, prompting proactive measures to cultivate a shift in attitude. By delving into the insights provided in this comprehensive guide and applying its principles, you pave the way to fortify yourself against stress and burnout. Embracing this journey involves a concerted effort to transmute negative thoughts into positive actions, a transformative process that, while demanding, yields invaluable rewards, promising a life enriched with newfound positivity and resilience.

"To be calm when others are not shifts the advantage to you in two ways:
—It stabilizes your position.
—It encourages allies impressed by your self-control."

9

MIND-BUILDING AND LIFE-BUILDING

James Allen

Everything, both in nature and the works of man, is produced by a process of building. The rock is built up of atoms; the plant, the animal, and man are built up of cells; a house is built of bricks, and a book is built of letters. A world is composed of a large number of forms, and a city of a large number of houses. The arts, sciences, and institutions of a nation are built up by the efforts of individuals. The history of a nation is the building of its deeds.

The process of building necessitates the alternate process of breaking down. Old forms that have served their purpose are broken up, and the material of which they are composed enters into new combinations. There is reciprocal integration and disintegration. In all compounded bodies, old cells are ceaselessly being broken up, and new cells are formed to take their place.

The works of man also require to be continually renewed until they have become old and useless, when they are torn down in order that some better purpose may be served. These two processes of breaking down and building up in Nature are called death and life; in the artificial works of man they are called destruction and restoration.

This dual process, which obtains universally in things visible, also obtains universally in things invisible. As a body is built of cells, and a house of bricks, so a man's mind is built of thoughts. The various characters of men are none other than compounds of thoughts of varying combinations. Herein we see the deep truth of the saying, "As a man thinketh in his heart, so is he." Individual characteristics are fixed processes of thought; that is, they are fixed in the sense that they have become such an integral part of the character that they can be only altered or removed by a protracted effort of the will, and by much self-discipline. Character is built in the same way as a tree or a house is built—namely, by the ceaseless addition of new material, and that material is thought. By the aid of millions of bricks a city is built; by the aid of millions of thoughts a mind, a character, is built.

Every man is a mind builder, whether he recognizes it or not. Every man must perforce think, and every thought is another brick laid down in the edifice of mind. Such "brick laying" is done loosely and carelessly by a vast number of people, the result being unstable and tottering characters that are ready to go down under the first little gust of trouble or temptation.

Some, also, put into the building of their minds large numbers of impure thoughts; these are so many rotten bricks that crumble away as fast as they are put in, leaving always an unfinished and unsightly building, and one which can afford no comfort and no shelter for its possessor.

Debilitating thoughts about one's health, enervating thoughts concerning unlawful pleasures, weakening thoughts of failure, and sickly thoughts of self-pity and self-praise are useless bricks with which no substantial mind temple can be raised.

Pure thoughts, wisely chosen and well placed, are so many

durable bricks which will never crumble away, and from which a finished and beautiful building, and one which affords comfort and shelter for its possessor, can be rapidly erected.

Bracing thoughts of strength, of confidence, of duty; inspiring thoughts of a large, free, unfettered, and unselfish life, are useful bricks with which a substantial mind temple can be raised; and the building of such a temple necessitates that old and useless habits of thought be broken down and destroyed.

> Build thee more stately mansions, O my soul! As the swift
> seasons roll.

Each man is the builder of himself. If he is the occupant of a jerry-built hovel of a mind that lets in the rains of many troubles, and through which blow the keen winds of oft-recurring disappointments, let him get to work to build a more noble mansion which will afford him better protection against those mental elements. Trying to weakly shift the responsibility for his jerry-building on to the devil, or his forefathers, or anything or anybody but himself, will neither add to his comfort, nor help him to build a better habitation.

When he wakes up to a sense of his responsibility, and an approximate estimate of his power, then he will commence to build like a true workman, and will produce a symmetrical and finished character that will endure, and be cherished by posterity, and which, while affording a never failing protection for himself, will continue to give shelter to many a struggling one when he has passed away.

The whole visible universe is framed on a few mathematical principles. All the wonderful works of man in the material world have been brought about by the rigid observance of a few underlying principles; and all that there is to the making of a successful, happy, and beautiful life, is the knowledge and application of a few simple, root principles.

If a man is to erect a building that is to resist the fiercest storms, he must build it on a simple, mathematical principle, or law, such as the square or the circle; if he ignores this, his edifice will topple down even before it is finished.

Likewise, if a man is to build up a successful, strong, and exemplary life—a life that will stoutly resist the fiercest storms of adversity and temptation—it must be framed on a few simple, undeviating moral principles.

Four of these principles are Justice, Rectitude, Sincerity, and Kindness. These four ethical truths are to the making of a life what the four lines of a square are to the building of a house. If a man ignores them and thinks to obtain success and happiness and peace by injustice, trickery, and selfishness, he is in the position of a builder who imagines he can build a strong and durable habitation while ignoring the relative arrangement of mathematical lines, and he will, in the end, obtain only disappointment and failure.

He may, for a time, make money, which will delude him into believing that injustice and dishonesty pay well; but in reality his life is so weak and unstable that it is ready at any moment to fall; and when a critical period comes, as come it must, his affairs, his reputation, and his riches crumble to ruins, and he is buried in his own desolation.

It is totally impossible for a man to achieve a truly successful and happy life who ignores the four moral principles enumerated, whilst the man who scrupulously observes them in all his dealings can no more fail of success and blessedness than the earth can fail of the light and warmth of the sun so long as it keeps to its lawful orbit; for he is working in harmony with the fundamental laws of the universe; he is building his life on a basis which cannot be altered or overthrown, and, therefore, all that he does will be so strong and durable, and all the parts of his life will be so coherent, harmonious, and firmly knit that it cannot possibly be brought to ruin.

In all the universal forms which are built up by the Great Invisible and unerring Power, it will be found that the observance of mathematical law is carried out with unfailing exactitude down to the most minute detail. The microscope reveals the fact that the infinitely small is as perfect as the infinitely great.

A snowflake is as perfect as a star. Likewise, in the erection of a building by man, the strictest attention must be paid to every detail.

A foundation must first be laid, and, although it is to be buried and hidden, it must receive the greatest care, and be made stronger than any other part of the building; then stone upon stone, brick upon brick is carefully laid with the aid of the plumb line, until at last the building stands complete in its durability, strength, and beauty.

Even so it is with the life of a man. He who would have a life secure and blessed, a life freed from the miseries and failures to which so many fall victims, must carry the practice of the moral principles into every detail of his life, into every momentary duty and trivial transaction. In every little thing he need be thorough and honest, neglecting nothing.

To neglect or misapply any little detail—be he commercial man, agriculturist, professional man, or artisan—is the same as neglecting a stone or a brick in a building, and it will be a source of weakness and trouble.

The majority of those who fail and come to grief do so through neglecting the apparently insignificant details.

It is a common error to suppose that little things can be passed by, and that the greater things are more important, and should receive all attention; but a cursory glance at the universe, as well as a little serious reflection on life, will teach the lesson that nothing great can exist which is not made up of small details, and in the composition of which every detail is perfect.

He who adopts the four ethical principles as the law and base of his life, who raises the edifice of character upon them, who in his thoughts and words and actions does not wander from them, whose every duty and every passing transaction is performed in strict accordance with their exactions, such a man, laying down the hidden foundation of integrity of heart securely and strongly, cannot fail to raise up a structure which shall bring him honor; and he is building a temple in which he can repose in peace and blessedness—even the strong and beautiful Temple of his life.

10

GOING THE EXTRA MILE

Napoleon Hill

Going the extra mile means rendering of more service and better service than you're paid to render, doing it all the time, and doing it with a pleasant, pleasing mental attitude.

One of the reasons why there are so many failures in the world is that the majority of people do not even go the first mile, let along the second one. If they do go the first mile, they usually gripe as they go along and make themselves a darned nuisance to people around them. I suppose you know the type. But it doesn't apply to any of you, because if you were like that before you got into this philosophy, you're going to get over it very fast.

I don't know of any one quality or trait that can get a person an opportunity quicker than to go out of his or her way to do somebody a favor, or do something useful. It's the one thing you can do in life without having to ask anybody for the privilege of doing it. Unless you form the habit of going the extra mile and make yourself as indispensable as you possibly can, the only other way you'll ever be free, and independent, and self-determining, and financially independent in old age will be by a stroke of good luck, a rich uncle or rich aunt dying, or something of that sort. I don't know of any way anybody can make himself or herself indispensable *except* by going the extra mile, by rendering some sort of service that you're not expected to render, and rendering it in the right sort of a mental attitude.

Mental attitude is important. If you gripe about going the extra mile, chances are that it won't bring you very many returns. Where do you suppose I get my authority for emphasizing this principle of going the extra mile? Experience.

I've watched the way nature does things, because you won't go wrong if you follow the way or the habits of nature. Conversely, if you fail to recognize and follow the way nature does things, you'll get into trouble sooner or later—it's just a question of time. There is an overall plan in which this universe operates, no matter what you call the first cause of that plan, or the operator of it, or the creator of it. There's just one set of natural laws, and it's up to every individual to discover them and adjust himself favorably to them. Above all, nature requests and demands that every living thing go the extra mile in order to eat, in order to live, and in order to survive. Man wouldn't survive one season if it were not for this law of going the extra mile.

Don't render a million dollars' worth of service today and expect to get a bank check for it tomorrow. If you start out to render a million dollars' worth of service, you might have to render it a little bit at a time. You're going to have to get yourself recognized for doing it and you'll have to go the extra mile for a little while before anybody takes notice of you. However, be careful not to go the extra mile *too* long without somebody taking notice of you. If the right fellow doesn't take notice, look around until you find the right fellow who will. In other words, if your present employer doesn't recognize you, fire the employer sooner or later and let his competitor know what kind of service you're rendering. I assure you it won't hurt your chances a bit. Have a little competition as you go along.

Nobody ever accepts a rule or does anything without a motive, and I have a great variety of reasons why you should go the extra mile.

THE LAW OF INCREASING RETURNS

The law of increasing returns means that you'll get back more than you give out, whether it's good or bad, whether it's positive or negative. That's the way the law of nature works. **Whatever you give out, whatever you do to or for another person, or whatever you give out from yourself, comes back to you greatly multiplied in kind.** No exception whatsoever. It doesn't always come back very quickly; sometimes it takes longer than you expect. But you may be sure that if you send out some negative influence, it's going to come back to you sooner or later. You may not recognize what caused it, but it'll come back. It won't overlook you.

The law of increasing returns is eternal, automatic, and it's working all the time. It's just as inexorable as the law of gravitation. Nobody in the world can circumvent it, go around it, or have it suspended for one moment. It's operating all the time. The law of increasing returns means that when you go out of your way to render more service and better service than you're paid to render, it's impossible for you *not* to get back more than you really did, because the law of increasing returns takes care of that. If you're working for a salary, the law takes care of it in additional wages, greater responsibilities, promotions, or opportunities to go into business for yourself. In a thousand and one different ways, it'll come back.

THE LAW OF COMPENSATION

It doesn't always come back from the source to which you rendered the service. Don't be afraid to render service to a greedy buyer or a greedy employer. It makes no difference to whom you render service. If you render it in good faith and in good spirit, and keep doing it as a matter of habit, it's equally impossible for you *not* to be compensated as it is to *be* compensated. Therefore, you don't have to be too careful about the person to whom you render it. In fact, apply this principle with *everybody*, no matter who it is—strangers, acquaintances, business associates, and relatives, too. Make it your business to render useful service to everyone, regardless of the shape, form, or fashion in which you touch them.

The only way you can increase the space that you occupy in the world—and I don't mean just the physical space, but also the mental and the spiritual space as well—will be determined by the quality and the quantity of the service that you render. In addition to the quality and the quantity, is the mental attitude in which you render it. Those are the determining factors as to how far you'll go in life, how much you'll get out of life, how much you'll enjoy life, and how much peace of mind you'll have.

SELF-PROMOTION

Self-promotion elicits the favorable attention of other people. If you're alert-minded and take notice, you'll find in any organization those people that are going the extra mile. You'll find out very quickly. And if you watch the procedure and the records of those people who are going the extra mile, you'll see that when there are promotions around, they're the ones that get them. They don't have to ask for them; it's not necessary at all. Employers *look* for people who will go the extra mile. It permits one to become indispensable in many different human relationships. It enables one to command more than the average compensation.

GIVING FEEDS THE SOUL

I want you to know that it also does something to your soul inside of you; it makes you feel better. And if there were no other reason in the world why you should go the extra mile, I'd say that would be adequate. There are a lot of things in life that cause us to have negative feelings or cause us unpleasant experiences and feelings. However, this is one thing that you can do for yourself that'll *always* give you a pleasant feeling. And if you'll go back through your own experiences, I'm sure you'll remember that you never did a kind thing for anybody without getting a great deal of joy out of it. Maybe the other fellow didn't appreciate it, but that's unimportant.

It's like love. To have loved, that alone is a great privilege. It makes no difference whatsoever whether your love was returned by the other person. You've had the benefit by the emotion of love itself. So it is by the principle of going the extra mile. It'll do something *to you*. It'll give you greater courage. It'll enable you to overcome inhibitions and inferiority complexes that you've been storing through the years. There is so much benefit available to stepping out and making yourself useful to somebody.

If you do something courteous or useful for somebody who is not expecting it, don't be too surprised when they look at you in a quizzical sort of way, as much as to say, "Well, I just wonder why you're doing that." Some people will be a little bit surprised when you go out of your way to be useful to them.

MENTAL AND PHYSICAL BENEFITS

Going the extra mile in all forms of service will lead to mental growth and physical perfection across all areas as well as greater ability and skill in one's chosen vocation. Whether you're delivering a lecture or making up your notebook, or filling your job, if it's something that you're going to do over and over again in your life, make up your mind that every time you do it, you will excel beyond all previous efforts on your part. In other words, become a constant challenge to yourself. See how quickly and how rapidly you will grow if you'll go at it in that way.

I have never delivered a lecture in my life that I didn't intend to deliver better than I did previously. I don't always do it, but that's my intention. It makes no difference what kind of an audience I have, whether I have a big class or a small class. I don't often have small classes, but when I do, I put just as much into a small class as a big one, not only because I want to be useful to my students, but because I want to grow and I want to develop. Out of effort, out of struggle, and out of the use of your faculties comes growth. It enables one to profit by the law of contrast. You won't have to advertise that one very much—it'll advertise itself—because the majority of people around you are *not* going to be going the extra mile, and that's all the better for you.

If everybody went the extra mile this would be a grand world to live in, but you wouldn't be able to cash in on this principle as definitely as you can now because you'd have a tremendous amount of competition. Don't worry. I can assure you you're not going to have it. You'll be in a class by yourself. There will be cases where people you work with or are associated with will be shown up for *not* going the first mile, let alone the second one, and they won't like that. Are you going to cry about that one and quit and go back to your old habits, just because the other fellow doesn't like what you're doing? Of course not.

It's your individual responsibility to succeed. That's your sole responsibility. You can't afford to let anybody's ideas, idiosyncrasies, or notions get in the way of your success. You can't afford to do that. You should be fair with other people, but beyond that, you're under no obligations to let anybody's opinions or ideas stop you from being successful. I'd like to see the person that could stop me from being successful. I'd love to see what he looks like, and I want you to feel that way about it, too. I want you to make up your mind that you're going to put these laws into operation and that you're not going to let anybody stop you from doing it. It leads to the development of a positive, pleasing mental attitude, which is among the more important traits of a pleasing personality—actually, not *among* the more important; it *is* the most important one. A positive mental attitude is the first trait of a pleasing personality.

It's a marvelous thing to know what you can do to change the chemistry of your brain so that you're positive instead of negative. Do you know how easy it is? It's as easy as getting in that frame of mind where you want to do something useful for the other fellow, without rendering service on the one hand and picking his pocket with the other. You're doing it just because of the goodness that you get *out* of doing it. You know that if you render more service and better service than you're paid to render, sooner or later you'll be paid for more than you do and you'll be paid willingly. That's the way the law works. That's the law of compensation. It's an eternal law, it never forgets, and it has a perfectly marvelous bookkeeping system. You may be sure that when you are giving out the right kind of service with the right kind of a mental attitude, you are piling up credits that'll come back to you multiplied, sooner or later.

UNLIMITED BENEFITS

Going the extra mile tends to develop a keen, alert imagination because it is a habit that keeps you continuously seeking new and more efficient ways of rendering useful service. The reason that's important is that, as you begin to look around to see how many places, and ways, and means there are in helping the other fellow to find *himself*, you find *yourself*.

One of the most outstanding things that I discovered in my research was that when you have a problem or an unpleasant situation you don't know how to solve, when you've done everything you know, and when you've tried every source you know of, and you're still at a stalemate, there is always one thing that you can do. I want to tell you that if you'll do that one thing, the chances are that you not only will solve your problem, but you'll also learn a great lesson. That one thing is to find somebody who has an equal or a greater problem and start where you stand, then and there, to help that *other* person. Lo and behold, it unlocks something in you. It unlocks cells of the brain, unlocking cells that permit Infinite Intelligence to come into your brain and give you the answer to the solution of your problem.

I don't know why that works, but do you know how I know that it *does* work? Do you know why I can make that statement so positive and not qualify it? I arrived at that decision by experience, by trying it out hundreds and hundreds of times myself, and by seeing it tried out hundreds and hundreds of times by my students to whom I have recommended that same thing. What a simple thing that is! I don't know *what it does* and I don't know *why it works*. There are a lot of things in life I don't know and there are a lot of things you don't know. There are also some things that you do know that you don't do much about. This is one of those things that I don't know anything about but I do something about.

I follow the law because I know that if I need my own mind to be opened up to receive opportunity, the best way in the world to open it up is to start looking around to see how many other people I can help.

PERSONAL INITIATIVE

Personal initiative gets you into the habit of looking around for something useful to do and going out and doing it without somebody telling you to do it. That old man Procrastination is a sour old bird and he causes a lot of trouble in this world. People put off things until the day after tomorrow that they should have done the day before yesterday. Every one of us is guilty of it. I know I'm not free of it and I know you're not, either. But I can tell you I'm freer of it than I was a few years back. I can find a lot of things to do now and I find them because I get joy out of doing them. Anytime you're going the extra mile, you're going to get joy out of what you're doing; otherwise, you won't go the extra mile. It will help you develop the quality of personal initiative and help you overcome the quality of procrastination.

Going the extra mile also serves to build the confidence of others on one's integrity and general ability, and it aids one in mastering the destructive habit of procrastination. It develops definiteness of purpose, without which one cannot hope for success. That alone would be enough to justify it. It gives you an objective, so that you don't go around and around in circles like a goldfish in a bowl, always coming back to where you started with something that you didn't start out with. Definiteness of purpose comes out of this business of going the extra mile. It also enables you to make your work a joy instead of a burden—you get to where you love it. If you're not engaged in a labor of love, you're wasting a lot of your time.

One of the greatest joys in the world is being permitted to engage in the thing that you would rather do than all other things. When you're going the extra mile, you're doing just exactly that. You don't have to do it, nobody expects you to do it, and nobody asks you to do it. Certainly no employer would ask his employees to go the extra mile. He might ask for extra help once in a while, but he wouldn't do it as a regular thing. It's something that you do on your own initiative, and it gives a dignity to your labor. Even if you're digging a ditch, you're *helping* somebody, and there's a certain dignity to that which takes the fatigue and the unpleasantness out of the labor.

Going the extra mile often gives the greatest amount of joy. You might think you go the extra mile being married, but what about before you get married? Believe me, I spent a lot of time burning midnight oil and I didn't consider it hard work at all. It was my own idea and I used my initiative, but I also got a lot of joy out of doing it and I made it pay off. When you're courting the girl of your choice (or being courted by the man of your choice), it's marvelous how much sleep you can lose and still not be seriously hurt by it. Wouldn't it be a wonderful thing if you could put the same attitude into your relations with people professionally or in the business that you put into courtship? We're going to start sparking again.

It's going to start at home, with our own mates. I couldn't begin to tell you the number of married couples that I've started in on a new sparking spree. They're getting a lot of joy out of it. It saves a lot of friction and a lot of argument. It cuts down expenses. Go ahead and laugh, but it will do you good.

I don't mean to be facetious. I'm very serious when I say that there is one of the finest places in the world to start going the extra mile. When you start going the extra mile with somebody that you haven't seen, sit down and have a little sales talk with them. Tell them that you've changed your attitude and you want a mutual agreement for both parties to change the attitude so that from here on out, *all* of us are going the extra mile. We're going to relate together on a different basis, where we'll all get joy out of it, more peace of mind, and more happiness in living. Wouldn't it be a wonderful thing if you went home tonight and had that kind of speech with your mate? It wouldn't hurt; it might help. Your mate might not be impressed by it, but you will be. Nothing will hinder you from enjoying it.

What about that person in business that you haven't been getting along so well with? Why not go in tomorrow morning with a smile and walk over to him or her and shake his hand and say, "Now look here and listen up, pal. From here on out, let's you and I enjoy working together." What would he say? It wouldn't work, huh? Oh, yes, it would. You try it and see. There's another thing that we have called pride, and if there's one thing that does more damage in this world than any other one, it's that little thing called pride. Don't be afraid. Don't be afraid to humiliate yourself if it's going to build better human relations with the people that you have to associate with all the time.

ESTABLISH OBLIGATION

Going the extra mile is the only thing that gives one the right to ask for promotions or more pay. Did you ever stop to think about that? You don't have a leg to stand on if you go to the purchaser of your services and ask for more money or for promotion to a better job unless, for some time previously, you have been going the extra mile and doing more than you're paid for. Obviously, if you're doing no more than you're paid for, then you're being paid for all you're entitled to, aren't you? Certainly, you are. So you have to first start going the extra mile and put the other fellow under obligation to you before you can ask any favors of him. And if you have enough people whom you have put under obligations to you by going the extra mile, when you need some favor, you can always turn in one direction or other and get it. It's a nice thing to know that you have that kind of credit hanging around, isn't it? I want you to have that kind of credit with other people and I want to teach you the technique by which you can do that.

NATURE GOES THE EXTRA MILE

We get our cue as to the soundness of the principle of going the extra mile by observing nature, and there's quite a bit of illustration regarding that. You will see that nature goes the extra mile by producing not only enough of everything for her needs but also a surplus for emergencies and waste. It shows this by the blooms on the trees and the fishes in the seas. She doesn't just produce enough fish to perpetuate the species; she produces enough to feed the snakes and the alligators and everything else. She produces those that die of natural causes, and even more, so there's enough to perpetuate the species. Nature is most bountiful in her business of going the extra mile, and in return, she is very demanding in seeing that every living creature goes the extra mile. Bees are provided with honey as compensation for their services in fertilizing the flowers in which the honey is attractively stored.

But they have to perform the service to get the honey, and it must be performed in advance.

You've heard it said that the birds of the air and the beasts of the jungle neither weave nor spin, but they always live and eat. If you observe wildlife at all, you'll see they don't eat without performing some sort of service, without working or doing something before they can eat. Take a flock of common old cornfield crows, for instance. They have to be organized in order to travel in flocks. And they have sentinels to protect them and codes by which they warn one another. In other words, they have to do a lot of educating before they can even eat safely.

Nature requires man to go the extra mile if he's going to have food. All food comes out of the ground, and if he's going to have food, he's got to plant seed. He can't live entirely on what nature plants (at least not in civilized life). On islands where they're not civilized, I suppose they depend on eating raw coconuts and what have you, but in civilized life, we have to plant our food in the ground. We have to clear the ground first before we plow it, harrow it, fence it, protect it against predatory animals and so forth. All of that costs labor and time and money. All of that has to be done in advance or you're not going to eat. I wouldn't have any trouble at all selling this idea that nature makes everybody go the extra mile to a farmer, because he already knows it beyond any question of a doubt. He knows every minute of his life that if he doesn't go the extra mile, he doesn't eat and he doesn't have anything to sell. A new employee can't start going the extra mile and immediately demand top wages or the best job in the place. It doesn't work out that way. You have to establish a record, a reputation. You have to get yourself recognized and received before you can begin to put the pressure on to get compensation back. If you go the extra mile in the right sort of mental attitude, chances are a thousand to one you'll never have to ask for compensation for the service you render, because it'll be tendered to you automatically, in the way of promotions or increased salary.

LAW OF COMPENSATION

Throughout the whole universe, everything has been so arranged through the law of compensation (and so adequately described by Emerson) that nature's budget is balanced. Everything has its opposite equivalent in something else. Positive and negative in every unit of energy, day and night, hot and cold, success and failure, sweet and sour, happiness and misery, man and woman. Everywhere and in everything, one may see the law of action and reaction in operation. Everything you do, everything you think, and every thought that you release causes a reaction, on somebody else or on you as the person releasing the thought. Because when you release a thought, you're not through with it. Every thought that you express, silently even, becomes a definite part of the pattern of your subconscious mind.

If you store in that subconscious mind enough negative thoughts, you'll be predominantly negative. And if you follow the habit of releasing only the positive thoughts, your subconscious pattern will be predominantly positive, and you will attract to you all of the things that you want. If you're negative, you'll repel the things that you want and attract only the things you don't want. That's a law of nature, too. Going the extra mile is one of the finest ways that I know to educate your subconscious mind to attract to you the things you want and to repel the things you don't want.

It's an established fact that if you neglect to develop and apply this principle of going the extra mile, you will never become personally successful, and you will never become financially independent. I know it's sound because I've had a great privilege that you haven't had yet, but you will have, in time. I've had the privilege of observing a great many thousands of people, some of whom applied the principle of going the extra mile and some of whom did not. I've had the privilege of finding out what happened to those who did and those who didn't. **And I know beyond any question of a doubt that nobody ever rises above the ordinary stations in life or mediocrity without the habit of going the extra mile.** It just doesn't happen. If I had discovered one case, just one case where somebody went on to the top without going the extra mile, I would say then that there are exceptions, but I am in a position to say there are no exceptions because I have never found that one case. I can definitely tell you from my own experiences that I have never had a major benefit of any kind in the world that I didn't get as the result of going the extra mile.

I want you to become self-determining, so you can do these things without the help of anybody. The payoff will come to you when you can go out and do anything in this world that you want to do, and regardless of whether anybody wants you to do it or whether they want to help you or whether they don't, you can do it on your own. That's one of the grandest, most glorious feelings that I know—that whatever I want to do, I can do it. I don't have to ask anybody, not even my wife. But if I had to ask her, I would, because I'm on good terms with her.

PEACE OF MIND

Here's a little item now that's not to be sniffed at: peace of mind that I got out of all those twenty years of going the extra mile. Do you have any idea how many people there are in the world at any one time who are willing to do anything for twenty years in succession without getting something back out of it? Do you have any idea how many people there are in this world who are willing to do something for only three days in succession without being sure they're going to get something out of it? You'd be surprised at how few there are.

We're looking at one of the grandest opportunities that a human being could possibly have, especially here in this country where we really can create our own destiny and where we can express ourselves any way we want. Speech is free, activities are free, and education is free. There's wonderful opportunity to go the extra mile in any direction you want to travel in life. And yet, most people are not doing it. I have seen a time when there were not so many people interested in the philosophy because they were prosperous. They were doing all right and they had no troubles to speak of. Today, almost everybody has troubles, or they think they do.

Do you know what I do instead of finding out what's wrong with the rest of the world? Do you know how I put in my time? I try to find out what I can do to correct this guy here. I have to eat with him, sleep with him, shave his face every morning, wash his face, and give him a bath now and then. You have no idea how many things I have to do for him! I have to live with the guy, twenty-four hours a day.

I put in my time trying to improve myself, and, through myself, I try to improve my friends and my students, by writing books, by delivering lectures, and by teaching in other ways. It pays off very much better than it would if I sat down and took the old newspapers and read all of the murder stories and all of the divorce scandals and everything that's blazoned across the pages every day. I'm still talking about this fellow Napoleon Hill, who didn't have sense enough to decline Andrew Carnegie's offer to work twenty years for nothing. His declining years will be years of happiness because of the seeds of kindness and help he has sown in the hearts of others.

If I had my life to live over again, I'd live it just exactly the way I have. I'd make all the mistakes I made. I'd make them at the time in life when I made them, early on so I'd have time enough to correct some of them. And that period during which I would come into peace of mind and understanding would be in the afternoon of life, not in the forenoon, because I couldn't take it. When you're young, you can take it. But when you pass the noon hour and you go into the afternoon, your energies are not as great as they were before. Your physical energy, and sometimes your mental capacity, is not as great. You can't take as much trouble as you can in your days of youth. And you haven't got so many years left to correct the mistakes that you made.

To have the tranquility and the peace of mind that I have today, in the afternoon of life, is one of the great joys that has come out of this philosophy. If you ask me what has been my greatest compensation, I would say that's it. There are so many people at my age, and even much younger than I, who haven't found peace of mind and never will. They never will, because they're looking for it in the wrong place. They're not doing anything about it; they're expecting somebody else to do something about it for them. Peace of mind is something that you've got to get for yourself. First of all, you've got to earn it. As to how anybody can get peace of mind, a few of you would be surprised where you have to really start looking for it. It's not where the average person is looking for it. It's not out there in the joys of what money will buy or out there in the joys of recognition and fame and fortune. You'll find peace of mind in the humility of the one individual's own heart.

Engage in at least one act of going the extra mile every day. You can choose your own circumstance, even if it's nothing more than telephoning an acquaintance and wishing him good fortune. You'll be surprised what'll happen to you when you begin to call up your friends that you have been neglecting for some time and just say, "You were on my mind. I was thinking about you, and I just wanted to call and say how do you do, and I hope you are feeling as good as I am." You'd be surprised at what that'll do to you and what it'll do to your friend, too. It doesn't have to be a close personal friend. It just has to be somebody you know. Or, maybe relieve a friend from duty for half an hour or so, or have a neighbor send over his children while he attends the movies, or do a little babysitting for one of your neighbors. If you're going to be at home anyway, with children of your own, maybe you know a neighbor who would like to get off and go down to the movies but can't get away from her children. The children may be noisy, and they'll probably fight with your children, but if you're a real diplomat, you'll keep them apart. She'll be under obligation to you, and you'll feel that you've really been kind by helping out somebody who otherwise wouldn't have had a little freedom. It'd be a nice thing for some of you people who don't have any children to say, "Why don't I come over and baby-sit for you while you go out? You and your husband can go on a little courtship. Let me come over and babysit for you while you go out to the movie or go to a show." You'll have to know your neighbors pretty well in order to do that. Certainly, most of you would have some neighbor that you could approach on some such basis, and they wouldn't think you were crazy.

It's not so much what you do to the other fellow. It's what you do to yourself by finding ways and means of going the extra mile in little ways. Did you know that both the successes in life as well as the failures are made up of little things? So little that they're often overlooked, because the things that make success are such small and seemingly insignificant things.

I know people who are so popular they couldn't have an enemy. One of them is my distinguished business associate, Mr. Stone. He always goes the extra mile and look how prosperous he is. Look how many people are going the extra mile for him. There are a lot of people who, if they didn't make good money working for Mr. Stone, they'd pay him a salary just to work for him. I've actually heard one say that he's become immensely wealthy himself working for Mr. Stone. He said, "If I didn't make money out of working for him, I'd pay him if I had to, just for the association with him." Mr. Stone's not different from you or me or anybody else, except in his mental attitude toward people and toward himself. He makes it his business to go the extra mile. Sometimes, people take advantage of that. They don't act fairly with him. I've seen that happen, but he doesn't worry about that too much. In fact, he doesn't worry about anything at all, period. He's learned to adjust himself to life in such a way that he gets great joy out of living and gets great joy out of people. Write a letter to some acquaintance, offering him encouragement. In your job, do a little more than you're paid to do, stay a little longer on the job, or make some other person a little happier.

11

THE JOY OF ACCOMPLISHMENT

James Allen

Joy is always the accompaniment of a task successfully accomplished. An undertaking completed, or a piece of work done, always brings rest and satisfaction. "When a man has done his duty, he is light-hearted and happy," says Emerson; and no matter how insignificant the task may appear, the doing of it faithfully and with whole-souled energy always results in cheerfulness and peace of mind.

Of all miserable men, the shirker is the most miserable. Thinking to find ease and happiness in avoiding difficult duties and necessary tasks, which require the expenditure of labor and exertion, his mind is always uneasy and disturbed, he becomes burdened with an inward sense of shame, and forfeits manliness and self-respect.

"He who will not work according to his faculty, let him perish according to his necessity," says Carlyle; and it is a moral law that the man who avoids duty, and does not work to the full extent of his capacity, does actually perish, first in his character and last in his body and circumstances. Life and action are synonymous, and immediately a man tries to escape exertion, either physical or mental, he has commenced to decay.

On the other hand, the energetic increase in life by the full exercise of their powers, by overcoming difficulties, and by bringing to completion tasks which coiled for the strenuous use of mind or muscle.

How happy is a child when a school lesson, long labored over, is mastered at last! The athlete, who has trained his body through long months or years of discipline and strain, is richly blessed in his increased health and strength; and is met with the rejoicings of his friends when he carries home the prize from the field of contest. After many years of ungrudging toil, the heart of the scholar is gladdened with the advantages and powers which learning bestows.

The business man, grappling incessantly with difficulties and drawbacks, is amply repaid in the happy assurance of well earned success; and the horticulturist, vigorously contending with the stubborn soil, sits down at last to eat of the fruits of his labor.

Every successful accomplishment, even in worldly things, is repaid with its own measure of joy; and in spiritual things, the joy which supervenes upon the perfection of purpose is sure, deep and abiding. Great is the heartfelt joy (albeit ineffable) when, after innumerable and apparently unsuccessful attempts, some ingrained fault of character is at last cast out to trouble its erstwhile victim and the world no more.

The striver after virtue—he who is engaged in the holy task of building up a noble character—tastes, at every step of conquest over self, a joy which does not again leave him, but which becomes an integral part of his spiritual nature.

All life is a struggle; both without and within there are conditions against which man must contend; his very existence is a series of efforts and accomplishments, and his right to remain among men as a useful unit of humanity depends upon the measure of his capacity for wrestling successfully with the elements of nature without, or with the enemies of virtue and truth within.

It is demanded of man that he shall continue to strive after better things, after greater perfection, after higher and still higher achievements; and in accordance with the measure of his obedience to this demand, does the angel of joy wait upon his footsteps and minister unto him; for he who is anxious to learn, eager to know, and who puts forth efforts to accomplish, finds the joy which eternally sings at the heart of the universe.

First in little things, then in greater, and then in greater still, must man strive; until at last he is prepared to make the supreme effort, and strive for the accomplishment of Truth, succeeding in which, he will realize the eternal joy.

The price of life is effort; the acme of effort is accomplishment; the reward of accomplishment is joy. Blessed is the man who strives against his own selfishness; he will taste in its fullness the joy of accomplishment.